NEUROENDOCRINOLOGY: A CLINICAL TEXT

NEUROENDOCRINOLOGY
A Clinical Text

MARY L. FORSLING, PhD,
Senior Lecturer in Physiology,
The Middlesex Hospital Medical School,
London

and

ASHLEY GROSSMAN, BA, BSc, MRCP,
Lecturer in Endocrinology,
The Medical College of St Bartholomew's Hospital,
London

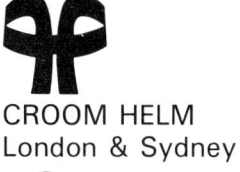

CROOM HELM
London & Sydney

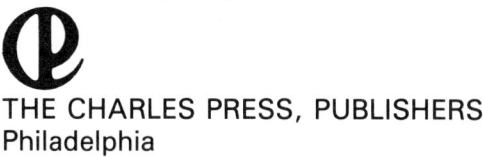

THE CHARLES PRESS, PUBLISHERS
Philadelphia

© 1986 Mary L. Forsling and Ashley Grossman
Croom Helm Ltd, Provident House, Burrell Row,
Beckenham, Kent BR3 1AT

Croom Helm Australia Pty Ltd, Suite 4, 6th Floor,
64-76 Kippax Street, Surry Hills, NSW 2010, Australia

British Library Cataloguing in Publication Data

Forsling, Mary L.
  Neuroendocrinology: a clinical text.
  1. Endocrine glands — Diseases
  2. Neuroendocrinology
  I. Title   II. Grossman, Ashley B.
  616.8   RC648

ISBN 0-7099-1041-X

and
The Charles Press, Publishers, Suite 14K,
1420 Locust Street, Philadelphia,
Pennsylvania 19102

Library of Congress Catalog Card Number: 86-7122

ISBN 0-914783-14-9

Filmset by Mayhew Typesetting, Bristol, England

Printed and bound in Great Britain by
Biddles Ltd, Guildford and King's Lynn

CONTENTS

Acknowledgements

1.	Introduction	1
2.	The Pituitary Gland	3
3.	Assays	13
4.	The Hypothalamus	31
5.	Control of Hormone Secretion	47
6.	Mechanisms of Peptide Hormone Action	62
7.	Prolactin	76
8.	Growth Hormone, Somatostatin and Growth Hormone Releasing Hormone	90
9.	The Gonadotrophins and Luteinising Hormone Releasing Hormone	108
10.	Thyrotrophin Releasing Hormone and Thyroid Stimulating Hormone	126
11.	Corticotrophin and its Releasing Factors	135
12.	The Posterior Pituitary	153
13.	Pituitary Tumours	173
14.	Neuroendocrine Test Procedures	190
Index		203

*To
Hannah and Alice;
Emily and Sophie*

ACKNOWLEDGEMENTS

We are very grateful to the clinical and scientific staff of both the Middlesex and St. Bartholomew's Hospitals. In particular, we would like to thank Prof. H.S. Jacobs, Dr C.G. Brook and Dr R. Stanhope of the Middlesex Hospital, and Professor I. Doniach, Dr J.A.H. Wass, Dr. R. Ross and Les Perry, Ray Edwards and George Piaditis of St. Bartholomew's Hospital, for their extensive advice and assistance. However, the final responsibility for the text must lie with the authors. It is in the nature of a rapidly advancing clinical science that many apparent facts are in fact speculative opinions, but we would hope that few would disagree with the majority of our interpretations.

1 INTRODUCTION

Since the pioneering work of Geoffrey Harris, studies on neuroendocrine systems have increased exponentially. This has been especially marked since the isolation and synthesis of the first hypothalamic hormone, thyrotrophin releasing hormone (TRH), in 1969. Fresh concepts have been developed to describe the relationships within the hypothalamic system and to study the pathophysiology of endocrine disease. New diseases have been described and those already known have become better understood, and the new discipline of clinical neuroendocrinology has come into being. There is now a vast literature on hypothalamic hormones in both animals and man, but this has been almost wholly confined to journals concerned with the basic science aspects of endocrinology and neuroendocrinology. This book is therefore aimed at providing an introduction to the expanding clinical science of neuroendocrinology.

It is now clear that there are releasing hormones for each of the major anterior pituitary hormones, and evidence exists for several release-inhibiting hormones. Secretion of adenohypophysial hormones is also influenced by feedback effects of the final products of pituitary hormone activity, occurring at both hypothalamic and pituitary levels, and neuroamine and neuropeptide modulators interact with the classical hypothalamic hormones. Certain of these interactions undoubtedly take place within the hypothalamic nuclei, but modulation at the axon terminals in the median eminence almost certainly occurs. The absence of axo-axonal synaptic structures at this locus suggests that classical concepts of information transmission within the CNS may require revision. There are intercellular contacts between different cell types within the anterior pituitary so that the output of a given cell may depend on the immediate environment. These paracrine interactions are assuming increasing importance, particularly in the gut, which may be considered as part of a widespread neuroendocrine axis involving information transfer and co-ordinated control. Even in the case of the posterior pituitary, long considered a simple 'output' from the supraopticohypophysial tract, recent research has suggested modulation of release by pituicytes. Finally, the spatial separation of the hypothalamic hormones in the median eminence, together with the spatial segregation of the portal vascular channels, indicates that our previous concept of an indiscriminate vascular pool transporting hypothalamic hormones to the pituitary urgently requires revision. Taken together, the discoveries of the last 15 years have led to a transformation in views concerning the hypothalamo-pituitary axis and to a greater awareness of its complexity.

These new insights are beginning to have extremely important consequences in clinical practice. Unfortunately, neuroendocrinology is perceived as something of a 'Cinderella subject' in medicine, and there is limited understanding of its concepts or usefulness outside of its immediate practitioners. Neuroendocrinology is often seen to involve arcane mysteries steeped in numerology and strange initials.

As neuroendocrine dysfunction is a common if underdiagnosed clinical problem, this is doubly unfortunate: first, communication between neuroendocrinologists and workers in other clinical specialties has become scrambled, and secondly, attempts at neuroendocrine assessment often seem to shed more confusion than light. Tests are sometimes used in inappropriate situations and their results are poorly understood. Like neurology before the age of the computerised tomography scan, neuroendocrinology is often left to its high priests. This attitude may be considered to be both unnecessary and unfortunate because, in spite of the increase in complexity of the subject, the basic principles are quite straightforward. Furthermore, the introduction of luteinising hormone releasing hormone and its analogues as therapeutic agents, and the imminent introduction of corticotrophin releasing factor as a diagnostic test and of growth hormone releasing hormone as a long-term treatment, require that all clinicians understand at least the basis of the subject. As a new clinical discipline, neuroendocrinology is based heavily on pure science and has few of the accumulated myths of some clinical disciplines to accept as received wisdom. It is crucially based on experimental biochemistry, although the overall concepts are few and relatively clear. This means that a good understanding of contemporary neuroendocrinology should involve a reasonable biochemical exploration of the basis of the subject, and we make no apology for the physiological/biochemical bias of an essentially clinical text. It is hoped that junior hospital doctors, senior medical students, specialists in non-endocrine disciplines and scientists and paramedical workers who come into contact with clinical neuroendocrinology will find this text a useful introductory guide. As clinical neuroendocrinology is one of the few clinical specialties that involve the whole organism and psychological as well as physiological aspects, we feel that it now deserves its own primer. We will have succeeded if we have indicated even some of the excitement of this expanding new clinical science.

Further Reading

Bennet, G.W. and Whitehead, S.A. (1983) *Mammalian Neuroendocrinology*, Croom Helm, London and Canberra/Oxford University Press, New York

Besser, G.M. and Martini, L. (1982) *Clinical Neuroendocrinology II*, Academic Press, New York

Martini, L. and Besser, G.M. (1979) *Clinical Neuroendocrinology I*, Academic Press, New York

2 THE PITUITARY GLAND

Introduction

Although the existence of the pituitary gland was known before the time of Aristotle, little information was available as to its role until the present century. Galen thought that the *pituita*, one of the four humors, passed from the brain and into the nasal cavity via the pallidum. Similar views were held by Vesalius who believed that waste material produced in the formation of the vital spirit was drained from the brain via the pituitary. This view was finally challenged in the seventeenth century by Schneider, who argued that the foramina in bone were for the passage of the olfactory nerves, and by Lower, who demonstrated experimentally that an increase in intracranial pressure did not result in passage of fluid to the nares. However, the true function of the gland was still unclear. Towards the end of the eighteenth century and the beginning of the nineteenth, it was argued that the gland was a large ganglion or, indeed, might be a replica of the cerebellum. Understanding of the true function did not really come about until the mid-nineteenth century when Pierre Marie noted the connection between acromegaly and the presence of a pituitary tumour, although he thought that the syndrome was due to hypopituitarism. Other disorders such as delayed puberty and obesity were similarly shown to be associated with pituitary tumours, but it was not until a successful technique for experimental hypophysectomy was developed that further advances could be made. Subsequently the activity of pituitary extracts was demonstrated. Evans and Long demonstrated the growth-promoting effects of pituitary extract, and Smith and co-workers showed its effects on the thyroid gland and gonads. Over the succeeding years the number of papers on the anterior pituitary has risen exponentially.

Understanding of the posterior pituitary stems from 1794, when Frank distinguished diabetes insipidus from diabetes mellitus. The activity of posterior pituitary extracts was established at the turn of this century. Schäfer and his team worked on the pressor and renal effects, and Dale described the uterine and Ott and Scott the milk-ejection activities of extracts of the posterior pituitary.

General Anatomy

The pituitary is located below the hypothalamus (Figure 2.1), hence the term hypophysis cerebri, derived from the Greek 'a growth under the brain' (*hypo*, under; *phyen*, to grow). The gland lies in a cavity of the sphenoid, the sella turcica (a picturesque comparison to a Turkish saddle), and is surrounded by the dura mater which lines the fossa. The diaphragma sella, a fold of the dura mater, separates the gland from the cranial cavity and has a small centre through which

4 The Pituitary Gland

Figure 2.1: Pituitary Gland and Surrounding Region in Man, Showing Gross Anatomical Features. The superior hypophysial artery supplies the median eminence.

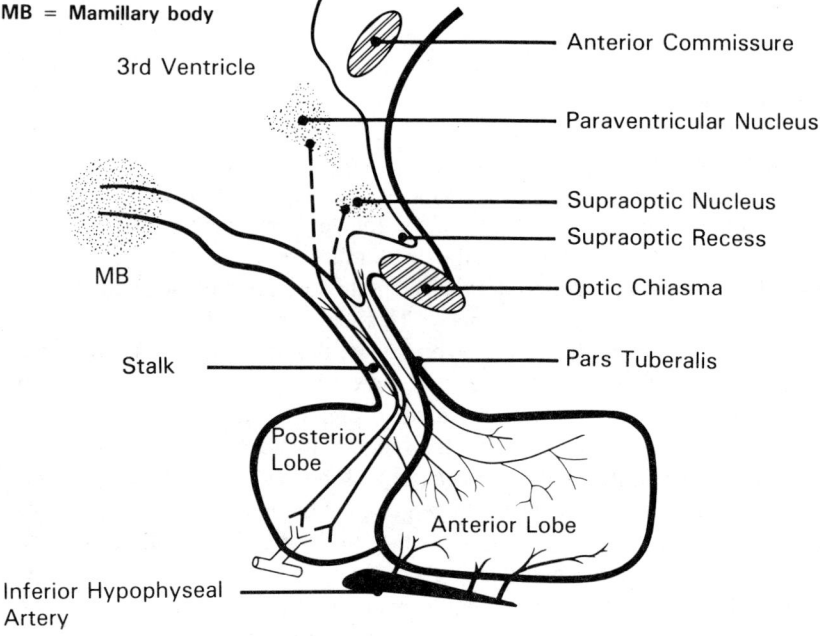

passes the pituitary stalk or infundibulum. The optic chiasma lies directly above the diaphragma sella in front of the pituitary stalk. The close anatomical relation to the optic chiasma is important, as compression by a spreading tumour may lead to visual defects. However, the precise position of the optic chiasma may vary, being relatively anterior in some instances (a prefixed chiasma) or relatively posterior (a postfixed chiasma). Hence field defects do not always correspond precisely to the degree of tumour extension.

The pituitary also has close anatomical relationships to a number of other important structures. Laterally are the cavernous venous sinus, the associated portions of the internal carotid artery, and the fourth, fifth and sixth cranial nerves. Anteriorly and below is the sphenoid sinus; this is usually an air-filled cavity, but is occasionally poorly aerated and thus relatively solid.

The gland itself weighs about 500 mg, and is slightly larger in the female, in whom, as Conte observed in 1898, the size increases during pregnancy and diminishes rapidly after delivery. The pituitary comprises two major components: the anterior pituitary constitutes about five-sixths of the pituitary, and the posterior pituitary the remainder. If a mid-horizontal section is made, the anterior pituitary is seen as reddish and kidney-shaped and the posterior lobe greyish; in a midsagittal section, the stalk is seen to bend sharply back to the posterior pituitary.

The terminology for the divisions of the pituitary as used by various authors is not consistent. The terms adenohypophysis and neurohypophysis include the pituitary stalk or infundibulum, which was not included in the older terms anterior and posterior lobes. Thus the term adenohypophysis is generally taken to include the pars anterior (pars distalis or glandularis), which comprises the major region of the adenohypophysis, the pars intermedia and the pars tuberalis or infundibularis, which surrounds the neural infundibular stem. The pars intermedia, which is distinct in most species, is not so in man. It is found as a rudimentary lobe in the fetus but virtually disappears in post-partum life. Recent work has demonstrated that there are a few scattered pars intermedia cells in the adult between the anterior and posterior lobes. There is some evidence for the presence of pars intermedia cells during pregnancy in the human, but it is rather insubstantial. The neurohypophysis includes the pars posterior, also called the pars nervosa or neural lobe, the infundibular stem and the median eminence.

Cytology of the Anterior Pituitary

The secretory cells of the anterior pituitary are arranged in irregular cords separated by vascular channels. These are larger than capillaries and are lined by endothelial calls, themselves held together in a reticular fibre framework. In 1886 two types of cell were described in the anterior pituitary, non-granular neutrophil chromophobe cells and granular chromophil cells. In 1892 Schoenemann further subdivided the latter into acidophils and basophils. Using conventional haematoxylin-eosin staining, the former are eosinophilic whereas the latter are more purple or cyanophilic.

These two cell types have a consistent arrangement in the normal human pituitary. Midhorizontal sections reveal that the acidophils are largely found in the posterolateral wings, while basophils are mainly in the median wedge and in the anterior and anterolateral sections of the gland. This spatial separation of the cells is important with respect to the localisation of microadenomas. In 1949 a great advance came when Pearse applied the periodic acid Schiff (PAS) histochemical method for the demonstration of glycoprotein to a study of the pituitary. It had already been recognised that the acidophils were associated with the production of growth hormone and also a pregnancy-related hormone. This was based on the observation that acromegaly was associated with tumours of acidophils and pregnancy with proliferation of acidophils. Now it was possible to identify cells containing the glycoproteins: follicle stimulating hormone, luteinising hormone and thyroid stimulating hormone (FSH, LH and TSH). Andrenocorticotrophic hormone (ACTH) -producing cells were also found to be PAS-positive, which was initially surprising as it was not thought to be a glycoprotein. However, it is now known that the N-terminal fragment of pro-opiocortin, which is co-secreted with ACTH, has a sugar moiety attached. The fact that the PAS-positive cells produced glycoproteins was confirmed by the observations on untreated myxoedema (hypothyroidism), and the findings in castrated animals when such cells were noted to increase in size and number. Many modifications of the staining technique were then applied to the investigation of the hypothesis that each hormone was secreted by a specific cell type. Using these techniques a number of secretory granules were identified, but unfortunately no uniform system of nomenclature was adopted.

More recently, the techniques of immunofluorescence and immunocytochemistry have enabled the site of synthesis of each hormone to be identified with a degree of certainty. These techniques involve the localisation of a specific hormone with antibody specifically raised to that hormone in other species. It is possible to visualise this antibody interaction by several methods. With immunofluorescence the antibody is linked to a fluorescent compound that can be seen by using the correct light source and filters. However, because of background fluorescence, the resolution of this technique is not very high, and the fluorescence tends to fade with time; it has therefore been little used for the pituitary. Other techniques involve the 'sandwiching' of several antibodies together to enlarge the macromolecular complex with an eventual enzyme-linked step to produce a visible product. Horseradish peroxidase is a commonly used enzyme in such systems.

Relatively few studies have been performed on the ultrastructure of the human adenohypophysis, but these, combined with studies on the rhesus monkey, are beginning to lead to the emergence of a clear picture. Although the early acidophil, basophil, chromophobe classification of pituitary cell types is a convenient shorthand for cell classification, it should be recognised that detailed analysis has now revealed at least five separate functional types.

Acidophils

The largest and most abundant of the acidophils are the *somatotrophs*, which are usually arranged in groups along the sinusoids. They are ovoid and contain large numbers of electron-dense spherical secretory granules 350–500 nm in diameter, and growth hormone is the secretory product. Prolactin is secreted by *lactotrophs* which are randomly distributed throughout the pituitary rather than mainly in the lateral lobes as previously thought. They are polygonal in shape but do not conform to a single morphological stereotype. In pregnancy there is an increase in their number. They have receptors for the steroids oestrogen and progesterone, as well as dopamine and thyrotrophin releasing hormone (TRH).

Basophils

Although classified here as basophils, the *corticotrophs* have occasionally been placed in the chromophobe category in subhuman species. They secrete ACTH and in the rat constitute approximately 16 per cent of cells. They are small cells grouped in clusters around the periphery of the central core of the gland, and their shape depends on the particular species. In man they are round or angular. They contain sparse secretory granules 300–350 nm in diameter. Following adrenalectomy these cells increase in size. Thyroid stimulating hormone (TSH) is secreted by the *thyrotrophs*, which form 2–4 per cent of the parenchymal cells of the anterior pituitary. They are elongated polygonal cells largely located in the ventromedial area of the lateral lobes. The granules they contain are irregular in shape and are only 100–150 nm in diameter. The number or cytology of the thyrotrophs is little affected by TRH, suggesting that this hormone mainly enhances exocytosis from the gland rather than *de novo* synthesis. In contrast, changes in the circulating concentrations of thyroid hormones produce marked changes in the number and staining characteristics of the cells, hypothyroidism resulting in an increase in the number of thyrotrophs whereas high concentrations of thyroxine lead to their regression.

The final group of hormone-secreting cells in the anterior pituitary are the *gonadotrophs*, responsible for the production of hormones controlling the gametogenic and steroid function of both the male and female gonads. They are larger than the thyrotrophs, are round or polyhedral in shape, and contain many dense granules approximately 200 nm in diameter. Considerable effort has been devoted to the differentiation of FSH and LH cells based on differences in staining, nuclear shape, distribution of granules, and changes following castration or FSH injections. More recently immunostaining techniques have been applied, but with the high concentration of antisera used, there is considerable cross-reaction between LH and FSH. Although it is held by many that LH and FSH are synthesised in the same cell in man, there is as yet no clear proof.

Chromophobe Cells

Very few chromophobe cells are apparent on electron microscopy of human pituitaries. In general, chromophobe cells are small with scanty cytoplasm indicative of low metabolic activity. It has therefore been suggested that they represent a non-secretory phase of the cycle of other glandular cell types. A further cell type is present in the colloid-containing acinar structures that lie between the secretory cells. These are elongated folliculo-stellate cells which form an intercommunicating network and hence have been ascribed a supportive and/or nutritive function.

Innervation of the Anterior Pituitary

Unlike the posterior pituitary, the anterior pituitary has virtually no nerve supply. The only nerves are a series of very fine nerve trunks which develop from the carotid plexus and follow the arterial branches into the anterior pituitary. They appear to serve a vasomotor function.

Pituitary Tumours in Relation to Pituitary Cytology

These may arise from any of the cell types just described, including the growth-hormone cells (10 per cent of pituitary tumours) and ACTH cells (5 per cent of pituitary tumours); the rest are either chromophobe or acidophilic. It is now known that about 40 per cent of the previously described 'functionless tumours' are in fact tumours of the prolactin-secreting cells. They stain with antiprolactin antiserum and are frequently packed with secretory granules. These true 'prolactinomas' tend to cause hyperprolactinaemia by direct tumour secretion of prolactin and are usually associated with very high concentrations of circulating prolactin.

However, many of the remaining tumours not immunostaining positively for prolactin may also cause hyperprolactinaemia by disrupting the portal vein delivery of dopamine to normal lactotrophs. In these cases serum prolactin is usually only moderately raised, but this is not invariably the case and serum prolactin alone is not an infallible guide to the differentiation between a prolactinoma and a functionless tumour.

Some studies have demonstrated that many of the functionless tumours may secrete the gonadotropins *in vitro*. It is possible that almost all pituitary tumours do indeed actively secrete pituitary hormones, but that in many cases these are not produced in sufficient quantities to modify circulating levels.

Growth hormone secreting tumours are associated with the clinical syndrome of acromegaly. Immunostaining often reveals prolactin cells scattered among the growth hormone cells, and these may occur in clusters. In some cases it appears that the prolactin cells are normal lactotrophs 'trapped' within the tumuor, and in others there seems to be a true mixed tumour of both lactotrophs and somatotrophs. Occasionally, cells in such tumours are found to secrete both growth hormone and prolactin, possibly suggesting that there is a growth hormone-prolactin cell precursor with the capacity to secrete both hormones. It should be noted that there is no clear correlation between the presence of hyperprolactinaemia (seen in 30 per cent of patients with acromegaly) and the presence of prolactin immunostaining within the tumour.

Tumours of the corticotrophs present as Cushing's disease. These are usually basophil adenomas but occasionally basophil hyperplasia is seen (this is very rare with other pituitary tumours). 'Silent' corticotroph tumours have also been reported.

All pituitary tumours are characterised by homogeneous sheets of cells compressing the surrounding tissue, but without a true capsule. The normal reticular network is disrupted by the adenoma and this may be revealed by special stains. Mitoses are uncommon, and malignant changes extremely rare. Although some degree of local invasiveness is not infrequent, true metastasis has very seldom been reported.

The Neurohypophysis

The neurohypophysis comprises thin non-myelinated nerve fibres terminating in neurosecretory nerve endings, which in turn abut on to vascular sinusoids. The perikarya of these neurones are the magnocellular neurones located in the supraoptic and paraventricular nuclei. For many years it was believed that the long axons passing from the supraoptic and paraventricular nuclei to the posterior lobe were the only oxytocin- and vasopressin-containing nerve fibres in the central nervous system. It has now been demonstrated that some fibres travelling from the perikarya in the hypothalamus are relatively shorter, ending in the median eminence and infundibulum. Fibres containing neurohypophysial hormones are also found outside the hypothalamus. In the infundibulum the nerve fibres are surrounded by astrocytes, but in the neural lobe 'pituicytes' form the bulk of non-excitable tissue. These are a type of glial cell, often with long processes, which lie parallel to the adjacent axons. Although they are mostly considered to have a nutritive function, recent work suggests that they probably contribute to the control of hormone release. On light microscopy the fibres are seen to contain 'Herring bodies' (or local expansions of neurosecretory granules) which electron microscopy reveals to be vesicles in the region of 200 nm in diameter containing the hormone precursor molecule. These granules are also seen in one type of nerve ending, the terminal axon endings which abut onto the fenestrated capillaries, which in turn receive the neurosecretions. These endings lie close to the sinusoids, although they remain separated by the basal laminae of the nerve endings and the pituicytes. Fine collagen fibres may also be found between the two. Also found in the nerve endings are smaller clear vesicles which probably arise through rupture of the synaptic membranes following secretion. Two other types of nerve ending are seen: periaxonal endings containing 80 nm dense core vesicles, and periaxonal endings containing small clear spherical vesicles, which synapse with the large hormone-containing endings. What interactions occur between these various nerve terminals is not known at present.

Pituitary Blood Supply

The arrangement of pituitary blood vessels and the direction of pituitary blood flow is of particular significance because of its relationship to the control of pituitary secretions. Our current concepts of blood flow through the pituitary are based on studies performed more than 50 years ago. Popa and Fielding found that the small parallel blood vessels running along the human pituitary stalk, and especially obvious in patients who had died following physical trauma, were indeed portal vessels, which when traced back ended in capillaries in the median eminence, and when followed downwards ended in sinusoids in the pituitary gland. Wislocki and King confirmed these observations, but the two groups did not agree as to the direction of blood flow in this system. The arteries of the pituitary gland arise as branches of the internal carotid artery, the inferior hypophysial artery which supplies the posterior lobe, and the series of superior hypophysial arteries which supply the median eminence and pituitary stalk. Two distinct capillary plexuses are present in the median eminence, an external or mantle plexus and an internal or deep plexus which arises from the external plexus. According to the classical concept of Wislocki and King, blood passes through the median eminence capillary plexus from which arise the long and short hypophysial portal veins through which blood passes to the secondary capillary plexus in the anterior pituitary. From there the blood drains through the systemic lateral hypophysial veins to the cavernous sinus. Blood from the posterior lobe drains through the systemic inferior hypophysial veins. Several modifications of this model have been proposed, the most recent being that of Bergland and Page who suggest that since the number and size of the lateral hypophysial veins appear inadequate to drain the anterior lobe, some blood crosses into the neural lobe. It is also suggested that an additional route for blood to leave the posterior lobe is through the neurohypophysial capillary bed to the median eminence from which it may pass rostrally to the hypothalamus. This reversed flow in the neurohypophysial system would provide a vascular route by which hormones released from the neurohypophysis could reach the hypothalamus and hence the CSF, and could exert a feedback control on their own release.

Recent work has suggested that the loops and tangles of the portal vasculature referred to as 'gomitoli' (Italian, meaning 'skeins') may have a topographical patterning such that specific regions of the median eminence are in specific contact with localised and equally specific areas of the pituitary. If this can be confirmed, it indicates that our views of portal blood passively transferring a homogeneous mix of hypothalamic hormones may need to be modified to allow for a more dynamic two-way flow of portal blood communicating between specific hypothalamo-pituitary zones.

Embryology

Rathke in 1838 described an invagination from the anterior end of the foregut (endoderm), but Balfour in 1874 and Mihalkovics a year later found that Rathke's pouch came from the embryonic buccal cavity and was ectodermal. In development Rathke's pouch differentiates to become the anterior and intermediate lobes of the pituitary. It is visible in the human fetus by 4 weeks. Rathke's pouch unites with the infundibulum which is formed as a result of the folding of the brain as an apparent outgrowth from the floor of the diencephalon forming the floor of the third ventricle, immediately behind the future optic chiasma. This eventually develops into the pituitary stalk and posterior pituitary. The front wall of the pouch thickens to form the anterior pituitary, and the back wall forms the intermediate lobe. A pair of lobes bud off from Rathke's pouch to form the pars tuberalis. A small remnant of Rathke's pouch is left behind in development to form the pharyngeal hypophysis, which is consistently present in the periosteum of the roof of the nasopharynx in man. By 18 to 20 weeks of fetal development in the human, the pituitary is capable of hormone secretion and is well vascularised. In the second half of gestation an extended trans-sphenoid portal system develops so that it comes under hypothalamic control.

Developmental abnormalities may occur during this process and persist into adult life. Thus rests of cells left over from Rathke's pouch may undergo metaplasia during early life to form the cystic tumours known as *craniopharyngiomas*. These usually develop from such cells in the suprasellar region, thus compressing the pituitary and optic chiasma below and the hypothalamus above, although they may occur within the pituitary fossa itself. They are usually partly solid as well as cystic, and frequently contain craggy foci of calcium. The cells are most frequently stratified squamous epithelium, lying in a loose matrix of connective tissue and often producing keratin, and the cysts contain a cholesterol-rich fluid resembling motor oil. Tumours composed entirely of stratified squamous epithelium have been termed epidermoid cysts, and those containing a wall of ciliated columnar epithelium have been described as Rathke's pouch cysts. However, it is possible that both are simply variants of the craniopharyngioma. These tumours will be discussed in greater detail in Chapter 13.

Occasionally the space in the arachnoid through which the pituitary stalk passes is excessively large such that changes in CSF pressure are transmitted to the fossa and herniation of arachnoid into the sella occurs. This increased pressure may gradually flatten the pituitary to a thin rim around the floor of the fossa: the 'empty sella syndrome'. In such cases pituitary function is generally well preserved, although mild interference with the portal vasculature may induce some degree of hyperprolactinaemia. The herniated arachnoid lining the fossa may occasionally 'round up', thus forming an *arachnoid cyst* within the sella. An alternative aetiology of the empty sella syndrome or of an apparent intrasellar cyst is infarction of a pituitary adenoma.

Neural control of endocrine secretion commences at least by midgestation in the human fetus, but is not complete until well after birth. The nature of investigations of human fetal endocrinology is obviously limited, but measurements have been made on tissue obtained at abortion or stillbirth, and several experimental animal models have been developed. It should be emphasised that caution must be observed in extrapolating from developmental observations on different species and on tissue obtained at surgery. By the eighth week after conception the diencephalon is differentiating in the human fetus, the ventral portion forming the hypothalamus. By 15 weeks the adult form of the hypothalamus has developed with all the nuclei differentiated. The supraoptic nuclei and supraoptic hypophysial tracts are present by the ninth week and neurohypophysial hormones can be demonstrated by the 12th week. An observation worth mentioning is that the amphibian hormone arginine vasotocin is found in the fetal pituitary of several mammalian species including man. Releasing factors have been detected by 15 weeks of development. There is little data on the ontogeny of putative neurotransmitters, but serotonin, dopamine and noradrenaline have all been shown to be present in the fetal hypothalamus by 12 weeks.

It appears that the three components of the hypothalamic-hypophysial portal vascular system (the primary plexus, the portal venous trunks and the secondary plexus) do not develop synchronously. The mature form of the portal system only develops in the second half of gestation, but it seems that there is functional interaction between the fetal hypothalamus and pituitary before there is complete development of this system. There is also evidence that this fetal hypothalamo-pituitary unit is largely autonomous of that of the mother.

The pattern of secretion of each anterior pituitary hormone develops differently in the fetus. The mechanisms of secretion of these hormones and their actions in the adult will be considered in some detail in later chapters, but a brief consideration of fetal hormones will be made here.

Control of growth hormone secretion appears to be immature at birth. Plasma concentrations of the hormone are high at 24 weeks' gestation and then fall away, but at delivery the cord blood concentrations are still elevated as compared with adult levels. The pattern of secretion is not significant in terms of fetal growth as the hormone does not seem to regulate somatic growth *in utero*; growth hormone deficient children appear to be fully mature and of normal weight and body proportions at birth. Similarly, prolactin probably does not exert any function in the higher mammalian fetus, even though the concentrations are high in the latter half of gestation in both fetal plasma and amniotic fluid. However, a role in the production of fetal lung surfactant has been suggested.

Prior to 26 weeks the activity of the hypothalamus and pituitary thyroid axis appears low. Between 18 and 25 weeks there is a marked rise in plasma TSH. The increased TSH secretion is reflected in a progressive rise in fetal thyroid hormones. The complete functional development of the thyroid appears to depend on TSH, although structurally thyroid growth is possible even in the total absence of TSH. There also appears to be increased sensitivity of the thyroid gland to TSH from 30 weeks' gestation onwards. Secretion of the other glycoprotein hormones, the gonadotrophins, is high in midgestation and decreases before parturition. The high levels probably reflect hypothalamic stimulatory influences, and the subsequent fall in secretion the development of negative feedback systems sensitive to sex steroids. Whereas fetal pituitary gonadotrophins in contrast to maternal chorionic gonadotrophin appear to play no obligatory role in sexual differentiation, they are necessary for growth and development of fetal gonads and external genitalia. Thus a boy born with deficient gonadotrophin function may have a micropenis.

The fetal pituitary has a rudimentary pars intermedia and the pattern of ACTH-related peptides appears to be different from those in the adult, although they still have only been poorly characterised to date. It is not known whether the fetal pars intermedia has a nerve supply; this is important as the fully functional rat pars intermedia is dependent on innervation for its activity. The fetal adrenal is also very different from that in the adult and it is suspected that it plays a role in the initiation of parturition. It is tempting to speculate that the fetal preference for secreting dehydroepiandrosterone sulphate rather than cortisol is controlled by a pars intermedia peptide. However, it has to be emphasised that such a peptide remains to be isolated.

Further Reading

Asa, L. and Kovacs, K. (1983) 'Histological Classification of Pituitary Disease', *Clinics in Endocrinology and Metabolism, 12*, 567–98

Doniach, I. (1977) 'Histopathology of the Anterior Pituitary', *Clinics in Endocrinology and Metabolism, 6*, 3–20

Flerko, B. (1980) 'The Hypophysial Portal Circulation Today', *Neuroendocrinology, 31*, 56–63

Lerner, A.B. (1982) 'The Intermediate Lobe of the Pituitary Gland: Introduction and Background', *Ciba Foundation Symposium, 81*, 3–12

Williams, P.L. and Warwick, R. (1980) 'The Endocrine System', in *Gray's Anatomy*, 36th edition, pp. 1437–44, Churchill Livingstone, Edinburgh

3 ASSAYS

Introduction

More than any other branch of endocrinology, neuroendocrinology depends on the use of sensitive and specific assays for peptides. It is generally held that the development of neuroendocrinology has progressed by quantum jumps as the isolation of each new hormone was rapidly followed by specific biochemical assays for its measurement in biological tissues and fluids. However, before the precise isolation and identification of these compounds, sensitive bioassays had detected the presence of important hormones. Thus, the first-named hormone, secretin, was identified by Bayliss and Starling on the basis of the measurement of biological responses, and not dissimilar techniques have recently led to the isolation of corticotrophin releasing factor (CRF-41) and growth hormone releasing hormone (GHRH). Nevertheless, bioassays are usually replaced in time by more structurally specific biochemical methods, most importantly binding assays which employ competition for a binding site, commonly an antibody (hence the widely used term 'radioimmunoassay'). There are also chemical assays, often employing chromatography with an on-line detector.

Bioassay

A bioassay or functionally-specific assay entails the determination of the potency of a drug (in the present discussion, a hormone) by noting its biological effect as compared with that of a standard preparation of defined activity. This type of assay is not routinely used nowadays, but played a vital role in the development of endocrinology and is still important in the standardisation of radioimmunoassays, particularly when hormones are not available in purified or synthetic forms as, for example, the gonadotrophins. In general, hormones are defined and named in terms of their principal activity, and when a radioimmunoassay, which detects a given chemical sequence, is established, it is necessary to correlate the results obtained with those from an existing bioassay. Failure to establish a close correlation between bioassay and radioimmunoassay has not always been a disadvantage and has led to some important discoveries. A case in point is pro-insulin. Radioimmunoassays for insulin yielded consistently higher results than those obtained by bioassay, indicating that there was in the plasma an insulin-like molecule with little biological activity. This eventually became known as the insulin precursor, pro-insulin.

14 *Assays*

Standards

Biological standards are generally extracts of the particular gland or of biological fluids. Their potency is expressed in terms of biological activity, i.e. international units (IU) per milligram of a given preparation. The earliest attempts at defining potencies were in terms of animal units. For example, the unit for steroids with androgenic activity was that amount which, when injected intramuscularly into capons, would produce a certain minimal degree of comb growth in a group of birds. This was the 'capon' unit. Many other such units existed. This was obviously unsatisfactory, so standard preparations were established and rigorous assay design was recommended. A large number of international standards and reference preparations have been set up which are intended as stable yardsticks against which the potency of other preparations may be determined. An international standard is a preparation for which an international unit has been defined on the basis of an extensive international study. This is not the case for an international reference preparation. An example of the former type of standard is the first international standard for arginine vasopressin, a synthetic peptide with an activity of 450 IU/mg which replaces the third international standard for oxytocin, vasopressor and antidiuretic substances, a powder prepared from bovine posterior pituitary. It is important to note that these units refer to a given response in a given system, e.g. pressor activity when injected into a rat, and that related hormones will possess different relative potencies in the various assay systems. Standards also have to be provided for radioimmunoassay.

There are a number of basic requirements for a bioassay:

(a) The unknown substance and standard must have the same action in the biological material that is being used in the assay.
(b) The responses must be obtained simultaneously (or nearly so), and matched biological material or preparations must be used.
(c) An assay must contain its own internal estimate of accuracy and reliability.

Bioassay of hormones may be performed using an intact animal, isolated tissue or a cell preparation. For the great majority (although not all) of endocrine bioassays, a plot of the log of the dose against the response yields a straight line. An exception to this rule is provided by the rat mammary strip assay of oxytocin, in which a log dose is plotted against log response. As will become clear, there are severe limitations to the number of observations that can be made in the preparation of the standard (stimulus-response) curve. When an assay is first established, five or six doses of the standard preparation generally indicate the linear portion of the log dose-response curve and will show the useful range of doses for future assays. Subsequently, in the execution of an assay, standard and unknown need only be administered in two or three doses each, the assay being defined in terms of the number of doses given. For example in a '2 × 2' assay two doses of unknown and two of standard are given. Sometimes only a single injection of unknown or standard can be given to any assay animal, so that many animals are needed. This applies to assays where one has to wait a number of days to observe the response, or if the process of observation itself is irreversible. Sometimes, when the response is fairly rapid, a preparation may be used repeatedly.

To gain some insight into the problems associated with the execution of a bioassay, several will now be described, examples being taken for hormones described in this volume. As will be seen, most bioassays are performed on that much-maligned but extensively investigated little animal, the laboratory white rat.

Assays in the Intact Animal

This type of assay has the advantage of monitoring the response in the whole animal, so that the activity obtained is likely to represent the true activity of the hormone. It is also more specific than, for example, assays employing an isolated strip of smooth muscle, which can give the same response to a multitude of agents. It has the disadvantage that, unless the manoeuvres involved are simple, such as an intraperitoneal injection, then the animal must be anaesthetised. Under these circumstances the response may be modulated by a number of factors, including the depth and type of anaesthesia and variations in blood pressure. In addition, if there is any likelihood that the endogenous hormone would be released during the course of the assay, then that particular gland must be removed or its hormone secretion suppressed. This is especially true of stress-related hormones such as GH or ACTH, the assays for which entail an initial hypophysectomy to remove the endogenous source. More recently, injection into the rat of antisera against both somatostatin and GHRH has allowed the animal to be used as a bioassay for ovine GHRH. Without such treatment, the results obtained are too variable to be of great value. Also, unless the injections are made into arteries directly supplying the target organ, the assay can be relatively insensitive because of dilution of the hormone in the extracellular fluid.

The Tibia Assay for Growth Hormone

This is an example of an assay in which a single response in one animal is observed. It is the most sensitive and probably the most reliable of the existing bioassays for GH and, although complex, is nevertheless the most convenient to carry out. Young rats are initially hypophysectomised under ether anaesthesia, four animals being used for each point. After hypophysectomy, the proximal epiphysis of the tibia rapidly decreases in width until it reaches a constant size some 12 to 14 days later. Daily injections of GH over the next four days stimulate chondrogenesis and lead to an increase in the width of the proximal epiphysis of the tibia, the width of the epiphysis being proportional to the amount of the total dose injected in the range 15–400 µg.

Antidiuretic Assay for Vasopressin

An example of an assay that entails repeated injection into the intact animal is the antidiuretic assay for vasopressin. Endogenous hormone secretion is suppressed by anaesthetising the rat with alcohol and giving it a water load. Once the animal is anaesthetised, the jugular vein and bladder are catheterised. Hydration and anaesthesia are maintained by means of an intravenous infusion of hypotonic saline and alcohol. The rate of urine flow is monitored using a drop recorder and the urine concentration is also continuously monitored. Injections of vasopressin produce an antidiuresis lasting some 10 to 15 minutes (Figure 3.1), so that repeated injections of hormone can be given over a period of hours. The degree of antidiuresis is proportional to the log dose, a response being obtained over the range 2.5–40 μU (approximately 6.25–100 pg).

Figure 3.1: Record of Traces Obtained for the Bioassay of Arginine Vasopressin (AVP) Performed in the Water-loaded Rat Anaesthetised with Alcohol. The upper trace shows the urine flow and the lower trace conductivity, which reflects the urine concentration. Injections of 5.0–40 μU vasopressin were given, which produced an increasing antidiuresis

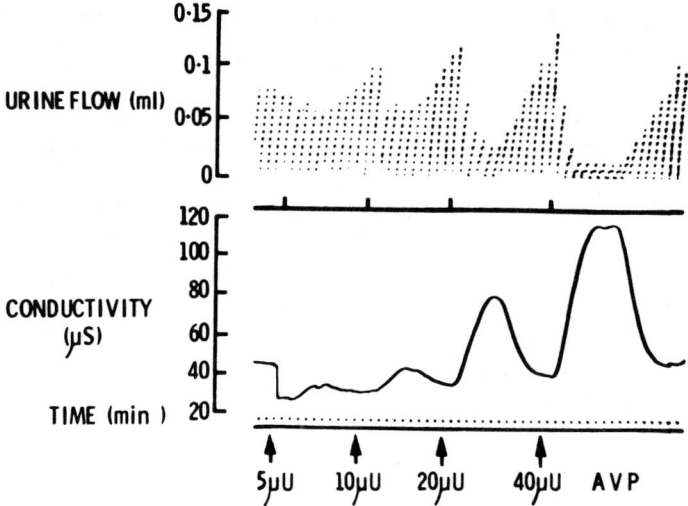

Isolated Tissues

Assays of isolated tissues have the advantage that they are relatively easy to set up and maintain.

Mammotropic Assays for Prolactin. These are *in vitro* assays in which single doses are applied to each tissue segment. Mammary explants from mice, rats or rabbits are incubated in synthetic culture medium for one or more days with insulin and corticosteroids. This permits morphological, but not functional, development of prelactating tissue. When prolactin is added, secretory activity is stimulated, and this can be evaluated histologically.

Mammary Strip Assay for Oxytocin. Lactating rats 6–14 days post-partum are killed, and small strips of mammary tissue are prepared and suspended in small organ baths of about 1 ml capacity. The tension developed by these strips is recorded using a very sensitive force-transducer. Application of oxytocin causes the strip to contract, the peak contraction recorded being taken as the response parameter. Repeated doses of oxytocin can be given, and a plot of log-dose against log-response yields a straight line over a dose range of approximately 5–250 μU (Figure 3.2).

Assays Using Cell Preparations

Cytochemical Assay for ACTH. In this assay the response to ACTH is assessed at the cellular level. The assay depends on the fact that the staining properties of the adrenal cortex are altered following application of the hormone. The exact biochemical reactions are unknown, but appear to relate to changes in adrenal ascorbate in the guinea pig adrenal zona reticularis. These changes are measured by staining with Prussian blue. It is a very sensitive assay as the immediate biochemical change is followed rather than the delayed physiological response. Furthermore, the hormone is applied to a relatively small number of cells rather than the entire tissue. The major disadvantage is the relatively high cost of the equipment and the difficulty of reproducing the results in different laboratories. This type of assay, although very sensitive, is in relatively limited use and is at present mainly used for the assay of trophic hormones. Guinea pig adrenals are divided into equal pieces and incubated in a synthetic culture medium for 5 h. The ACTH-containing sample is then poured over the adrenal tissue and is left for 4 min. The material is frozen to $-70\,^{\circ}$C, sectioned in a cryostat, and stained with Prussian blue. The depth of the staining is proportional to the concentration of ACTH added; in the presence of low concentrations of ACTH the staining is very dense and vice versa. The intensity of the staining is then measured using a scanning and integrating microdensitometer.

One major advantage of the cytochemical assays is their often exceptional sensitivity. Thus they are used, for example, to detect small changes in ACTH and parathyroid hormone (PTH) in the region undetectable by radioimmunoassay. For example, in certain patients with adrenal tumours, ACTH concentrations may be undetectable by radioimmunoassay but are readily measurable by cytochemical assay. This suggests that corticosteroids may limit, rather than totally inhibit, pituitary ACTH release, and the technique allows more refined investigations of steroidal feedback to be carried out. With regard to PTH, since existing routine immunoassays are not always very reliable, even in simply diagnosing primary hyperparathyroidism, the cytochemical assay may prove useful in this context. Such an assay is also at present in extensive use in the investigation of the non-peptide putative 'natriuretic hormone'. However, it should be emphasised that the cytochemical assay is highly dependent on the purity of the standards used, and, in addition, is precisely contingent upon accurate measurements of time as the reactions are usually quite rapid.

Assay Design and Estimation of Potency

As can be seen, considerable effort is necessary to obtain even a single

Figure 3.2: Record Showing Changes in the Tension of Rat Mammary Strip Preparation to Decreasing Doses of Oxytocin. The lower section of the figure illustrates a dose-response curve prepared using the trace illustrated in the upper section

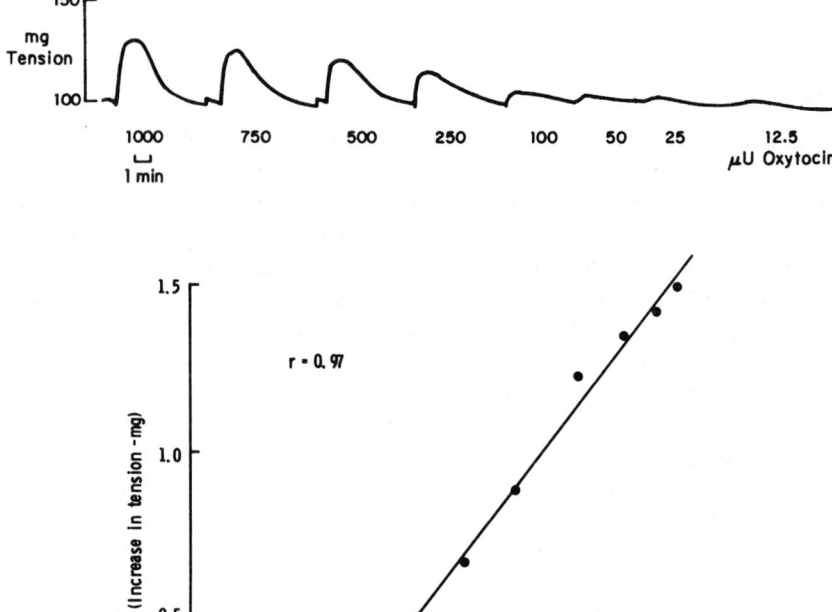

measurement on a dose-response curve. Careful assay design and analysis of results is essential. A four-point design (2 × 2) is commonly adopted for hormone assays, using two doses each of standard and unknown — a low and a high dose in the same ratio, frequently two, for both unknown and standard. This design does not allow the linearity of the response to be determined, but, and which is more important, does allow a check of the parallelism of the lines for standard and unknown. Parallelism indicates that the standard and unknown solution have given the same response in the assay preparation. For example, in the antidiuretic assay for vasopressin, acetylcholine could produce an antidiuresis by causing a fall in blood pressure. However, when the dose is doubled, it is most unlikely that acetylcholine and vasopressin would produce identical changes in the antidiuresis, and thus the dose-response curves would not be parallel.

A possibly more-satisfactory assay design is the 2 × 3 design in which standard and unknown are explored at three dose levels. This allows a check of parallelism and linearity. In special circumstances in which very little of the substance under investigation is available, a bracket assay may be used in which a single injection is bracketed by two standards. Formulae are available to determine the precision of any assay, producing the index of precision or the fiducial limits. It can be seen that the use and assessment of bioassays has needed a high level of sophistication, mainly based on research in pharmacology. However, the general trend in endocrinology is away from bioassays and towards saturation analysis.

Structurally Specific Assays

Within the last two decades a number of new microanalytical methods for the analysis of biological materials have been developed. All the techniques involve the combination of two materials, one of which is referred to as the 'binder' and the other as the ligand. The terminology relating to these assays can be confusing, but a term which embraces the whole field is 'binding assays'. An alternative title is 'saturation analysis'. This encompasses any procedure in which quantitation of a given substance depends on the progressive saturation of a specific binder by that substance, and entails the subsequent determination of the proportion which is not bound, i.e. which is in the 'free' phase. The most commonly used classification of binding assays is based on the nature of the binder employed: 'immunoassays', which use an antibody; 'competitive protein binding assays', using a naturally occurring binding protein; and 'receptor' assays, in which the binder is a naturally occurring cell receptor.

The determination of the distribution of ligand between the bound and free phases usually depends on physico-chemical separation, the distribution being followed by the incorporation of a 'tracer' consisting of a small amount of labelled ligand (usually radioactive), thereby giving rise to the term 'radioimmunoassay' (RIA). The use of isotopes is not a prerequisite of binding assays. Fluorimetric (fluoroimmunoassay, FIA) or enzymatic (enzyme immunoassay, EIA) techniques could be employed. It is also possible to use a labelled *binder* as tracer rather than labelled ligand, hence the term 'immunometric assay'.

Binding Assays

The principles of binding assays are simple. Although, in this chapter, radio-immunoassay will be used as an example, the principles illustrated apply equally to all systems under the general heading of binding assay. If given, fixed amounts of antigen and antibody are allowed to react together, then at equilibrium they will form an antigen-antibody complex, a proportion of the antigen and antibody remaining free (Figure 3.3). If the antibody concentration is held constant while the total amount of antigen is increased, then at equilibrium more of the antigen

20 *Assays*

will be 'free'. The concentration of ligand in the unknown sample ('x' in Figure 3.4) can then be calculated from a standard curve where the distribution between bound and free ligand is calculated for a set of standards with the same fixed concentration of ligand and antibody. The radioactive count 'y' then designates a certain concentration 'x'.

Figure 3.3: Diagram Illustrating the Basic Principles of a Saturation Assay. At low concentration of antigen (A), most of the radioactivity is in the bound fraction

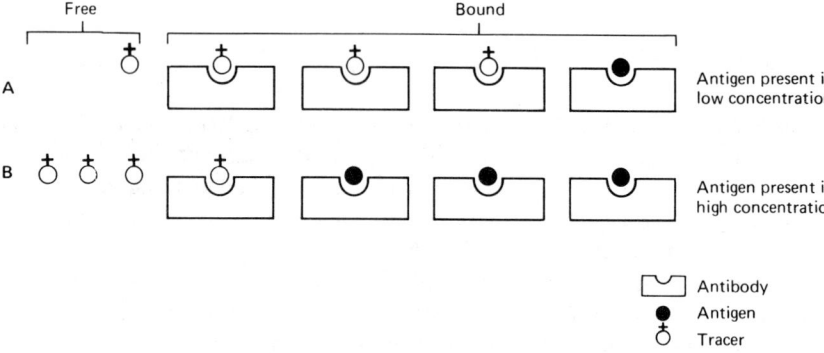

This type of assay has various requirements, notably: a specific binding protein of high affinity for the ligand; a pure preparation of the ligand to act as standard and for preparing a labelled derivative; and a means of separating antibody-bound and free ligand. The one assumption is that the labelled and unlabelled antigen have equal affinity for the antibody.

Binding Reagent

The binding reagent (either antibody or binding protein) should exhibit a high affinity and be specific for the antigen. Binding reagent specificity should not be confused with cross-reactivity. An antibody on testing may not cross-react with related substances, but only rarely has a comprehensive selection been used, and when the antibody is used in routine conditions the result may be higher than predicted. This may also be due to a number of effects including interfering substances in serum unrelated to the peptides being measured. This degree of interference is often unavoidable since most binding proteins exhibit some degree of affinity for related substances. The extent of the misclassification will depend upon the affinity and concentration of the interfering substances. For example, antisera raised against thyroxine (T_4) exhibit some cross-reaction to triiodothyronine (T_3), but the concentration of T_3 in most biological samples is approximately 100-fold lower than the T_4 and does not normally result in a significant error.

Labelled-hormone Preparation

The tracer may serve both as recovery indicator and as the indicator of the

Figure 3.4: Idealised Standard Curve for a Radioimmunoassay. The concentration x of a substrate can be determined by reading off its radioactivity count y from the curve. The standards are usually prepared in duplicate

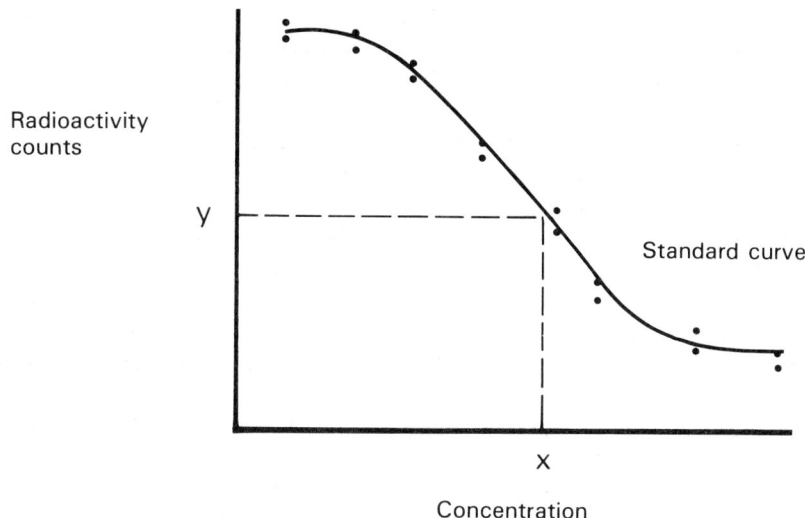

distribution of the free and bound moieties in the assay. Alternatively, a separate label may be used for each in the assay.

For proteins and peptides the label is generally prepared by reacting the substance with an iodine isotope (usually ^{125}I) and purifying the labelled product by gel filtration. In this case, the radioiodine is introduced into tyrosine or histidine residues. Another method, particularly useful for steroids and for proteins, and for peptides not possessing tyrosine or histidine residues, comprises conjugating the substance of interest to a compound that is already labelled. Tritium is also used extensively for labelling, particularly for small molecules such as steroids and cyclic nucleotides.

Three factors influence the quality of the labelled antigen:

(1) 'Radiolysis', where too many radioactive iodine atoms are incorporated into the antigen with the result that the radiation energy breaks the weaker chemical bonds. This leads to the production of radioactive fragments of the antigen with little or no immunoreactivity.
(2) Conformation of the labelled antigen can be changed if the purification step is incomplete during preparation.
(3) Incubation damage from incorrect storage or from the presence of proteolytic enzymes in serum samples.

Separation of Bound from Free Hormone

Ideally, the separation procedure should completely separate the bound and free fractions, and should be unaffected by variations in the constituents of the incubation mixture. These requirements are rarely completely achieved. It can be readily seen that all incubation mixtures (samples and standards) should be as near identical as possible, and differ only in the amount of the substance being assayed. For this reason, if unextracted plasma is being assayed, standards should be prepared in hormone-free serum. The separation is most usually achieved by either physical means (i.e. adsorption of the unbound on to talc or charcoal, or of the bound on to filters), or by precipitation of the bound (by ammonium sulphate or polyethyleneglycol), or by immunological means (e.g. using a second, precipitating, antiserum to precipitate the bound fraction). The separation step can be made simpler by using a solid-phase system in which the binding reagent is either physically bound or chemically linked to particles such as cellulose microbeads, or even to the walls of the incubation tube. The separation step, in these circumstances, then only requires centrifugation or decantation. A further advantage of this system is that the bound fraction can be washed, removing more completely the unbound hormone, so limiting the misclassification errors that occur in most assays.

There is little doubt that saturation assays have revolutionised the measurement of hormones, drugs, and enzymes, and there are few substances that have escaped its attention. It should be realised, however, that the antisera used are usually a mixture of immunoglobulins, each with a slightly different affinity for the index compound. Monoclonal antibodies are now available with a single molecular profile, and these may be more precisely tailored to different regions of the molecular species investigated. Nevertheless, for most routine purposes this degree of sophistication is unnecessary. Furthermore, it may actually be counterproductive to use monoclonal antibodies as there is evidence that many circulating peptide hormones constitute an array of related but distinctive molecular species.

Excess Reagent Assays (Immunoradiometric Assays)

This type of assay differs in principle from the saturation assays. The method is based on the addition of excess labelled binding reagent (usually an antibody) to the hormone being assayed. Following the reaction, the labelled antibody not bound is removed by incubation with an immunoabsorbent consisting of the antigen linked to cellulose or similar material, and the radioactivity remaining is determined. The same immunoabsorbent is used in the procedure for labelling the antibody. Serum from immunised animals is incubated with the specific immunoabsorbent and the antibody : immunoabsorbent complex is isolated and labelled, usually with ^{125}I. The labelled antibody is eluted from the complex by treatment with dilute HCl or other dissociating agents.

It is also possible to use a 'sandwich' assay in which an unlabelled antibody bound to the walls of a plastic tube reacts with the antigen and a second antibody (labelled) is then reacted. The excess labelled antibody left after the reaction is removed by simple decantation and washing. As the tubes can all be prepared in advance, this type of assay is obviously useful in obtaining rapid, reasonably accurate results with the minimum of technical expertise.

A variation on this method is to use alternative labels, e.g. fluorescein- or enzyme-labelled antibody. One such assay comprises the attachment of antibody (unlabelled) on the base of a multiwell plastic plate (96 wells). To each well is added the substance to be assayed followed by a second (enzyme-labelled) antibody. Following washing, the substrate of the enzyme is added and the extent of enzymic action is observed. Normally, a reaction is used that produces a coloured product. A further variation can be introduced in which the second antibody is not itself labelled but a further labelled antibody against the second antibody is used. Although this adds to the complexity of the system, it is a more universal system, and is much used in immunostaining.

In order to understand the problems associated with the performance of a saturation analysis, examples of each of the various forms of the assay will be described: direct immunoassays, an extracted immunoassay, and an excess reagent assay.

An Example of a Direct Radioimmunoassay

Most of the RIAs in common use are direct. These are relatively rapid, usually take 1 to 3 days, and are fairly straightforward to carry out. As an example, serum prolactin is usually measured by direct RIA (Figure 3.5). One protocol requires 50 µl of sample, to which is added 350 µl of diluent and a 50 µl aliquot of labelled prolactin. Prolactin is labelled with ^{125}I, and the freeze-dried preparation is stored in aliquots for convenience. Antiserum to human prolactin is raised in rabbits, and 50 µl aliquots of this are then also added. The mixture is allowed to equilibrate for 24 h; standards are also included. The sample prolactin and labelled prolactin partition themselves between free and bound phases, and at 24 h a second antiserum (raised in donkeys against rabbit immunoglobulin) is added. A further 24-h incubation allows the donkey serum to precipitate out all rabbit serum. After centrifugation, the supernatant may then be aspirated, leaving a precipitate at the bottom of the tube. The radiation counts per tube will then be proportional to the amount of labelled prolactin bound to the rabbit antibody; this will be reduced as the quantity of prolactin in the sample increases. Several controls are necessary to account for non-specific binding of the antisera, trapping of radioactive label, etc., and it is usual to include several samples of known prolactin content in each assay. This allows not only quality control to be carried out within the laboratory, but also different national laboratories to compare their precisions. Comparison of the radiation count of a given sample with values on the standard curve allows the serum prolactin to be determined. In the UK this is usually given in terms of mU/litre, with most laboratories giving an upper limit of normal range in men and non-pregnant women as 360 mU/litre. In Europe and the United States, values are related to a pure prolactin preparation, and are given as ng/ml or µg/litre (these can be numerically converted to mU/litre by multiplication by 20, i.e. 18 ng/ml = 360 mU/litre).

Samples are normally assayed in duplicate, and the mean of the duplicates

Figure 3.5: Scheme for a Standard Radioimmunoassay Using a Second Antibody

STANDARD RIA

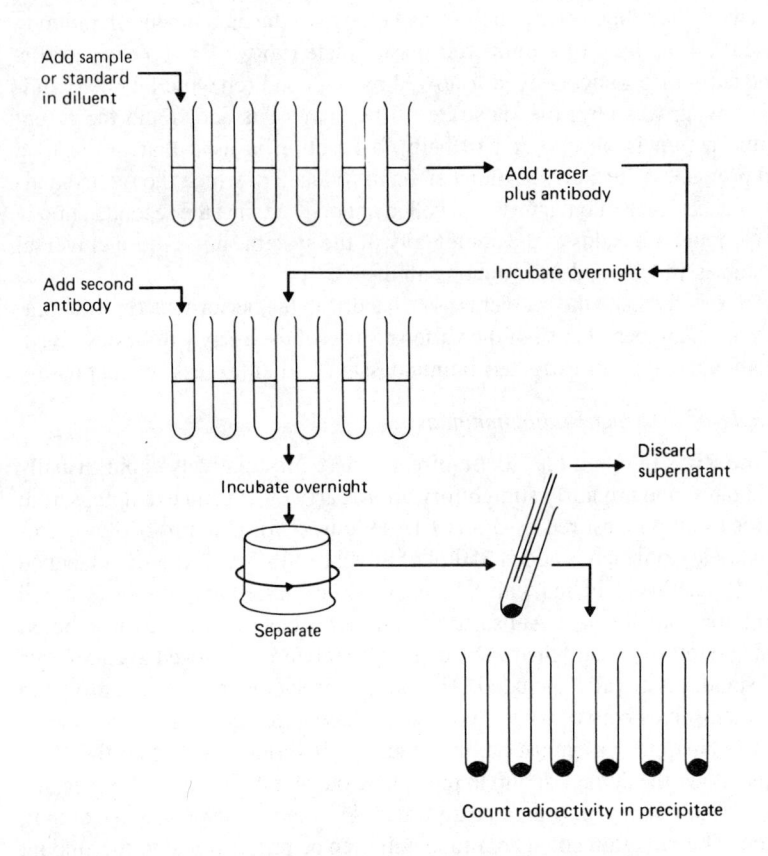

Add sample or standard in diluent

Add tracer plus antibody

Incubate overnight

Add second antibody

Incubate overnight

Separate

Discard supernatant

Count radioactivity in precipitate

is taken as the final figure. However, if the duplicates are different (> 5 per cent difference in counts), it is good practice to reassay the sample.

If a single sample of serum is separated into several aliquots and each is then individually assayed, a distribution or scatter of prolactin values is obtained. The standard deviation of this distribution, divided by the mean value, obviously represents the precision of the assay, and when represented as a percentage is referred to as the *coefficient of variation* (CV) of the assay. In clinical practice, serum prolactin for a given patient may be measured on several occasions, and hence in different assays, and thus the *inter*-assay CV is relevant. This is usually below 5 per cent, and should generally be less than 10 per cent for direct assays.

Although the assay has been described in detail for prolactin, broadly similar direct RIAs are routinely available for GH, LH, FSH, and TSH. There are obviously a number of variations in this procedure. For example, for some protein hormones such as TSH, the normal range lies in the area of the lower detection limit. If a preincubation is performed, during which the antibody and unlabelled hormone can combine and *then* the label is added ('late addition'), one can increase the sensitivity of the system.

An Example of an Extracted Radioimmunoassay

It is sometimes necessary to extract (or perhaps purify) the substances to be measured from the biological samples. Extraction may also be necessary if the substance to be assayed is bound to a protein in the sample (e.g. serum binding protein), or if compounds are present that affect either the reaction between the substance and the binding reagent or the separation step. Extraction is also necessary if the substance is present in such low concentrations that it needs concentrating. If extraction and purification are necessary, the recovery of the substance may be monitored by estimating the recovery of 'cold' hormone added to hormone-free plasma, or of a radioactive tracer added at the beginning of the extraction procedure.

Examples of immunoassays involving an extraction step are those for ACTH (Figure 3.6), vasopressin and oxytocin. Extraction techniques for saturation analysis are frequently based on those used for bioassay, being modified to allow a greater throughput. In the assay of vasopressin, the plasma is first acidified. This inactivates enzymes which could destroy the hormone, and dissociates what little hormone may be protein bound. The vasopressin is then adsorbed on to a silicate, such as Spherosil XOA or bentonite, a process also enhanced in the presence of acid. The adsorbent is then washed and the hormone is eluted with acetone/water or acetone/HCl. This eluate should contain a pure extract of the hormone dissolved in the organic solvent mixture. The solvent is then completely evaporated, and the remaining material is redissolved in assay buffer. A recent advance is the use of a solid column of silicate to adsorb to hormone, commercially known as 'Sep Packs'. The extract is then assayed in the normal manner. As the extract contains virtually none of the original plasma constituents, there are few factors to interfere with the hormone-antibody binding or the separation step. Nevertheless, 'recovery plasmas' with known amounts of hormone should be included in the assay.

An Example of an Excess Reagent Assay

A typical assay in this category is that for TSH (Figure 3.7). Anti-TSH antibody (e.g. sheep antibody) is linked to a solid phase, and is mixed with ^{125}I-labelled TSH antibody which binds to a different part of the TSH molecule; 400 μl of this mixture is added to 100 μl of the sample. All the TSH in the sample binds to *both* solid phase and labelled antibody to form a 'sandwich' with TSH as the filling; the amount of labelled antibody that is present in the solid phase indicates the amount of TSH in the sample. As TSH concentration increases in the sample, so does the amount of labelled antibody associated with the solid phase.

As opposed to conventional radioimmunoassay, which takes 24–48 h, this excess reagent assay may be performed in 3 h. Furthermore, it has a very wide working range; very low levels of TSH may be measured, as well as very high

26 *Assays*

Figure 3.6: Scheme for a Radioimmunoassay Employing an Extraction Step, Using ACTH as an Example

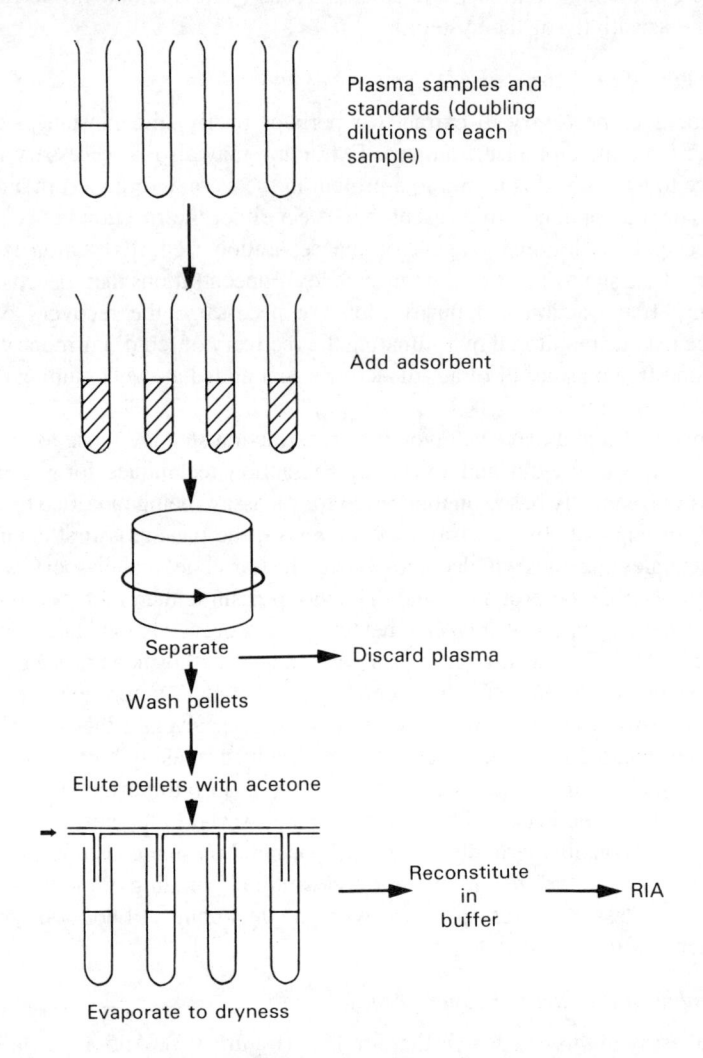

Plasma samples and standards (doubling dilutions of each sample)

Add adsorbent

Separate → Discard plasma

Wash pellets

Elute pellets with acetone

Evaporate to dryness

Reconstitute in buffer → RIA

levels without sample dilution. Conventional RIA cannot define the lower limit of the normal range, such that TSH levels less than 1 mU/litre may either represent thyrotoxicosis or normality. It is probable that this newer type of assay will allow this differentiation to be made on a single TSH sample. However, against the speed and sensitivity of this assay must be set its greater expense.

A second interesting use of the immunoradiometric (IRMA) assay is being developed in the measurement of ACTH. Conventional RIA uses antisera directed against just one part of the ACTH molecule, such that larger forms of ACTH (as exist, for example, in the ACTH precursor) are also measured. As the IRMA attaches antibodies to *both* ends of the ACTH molecule, the N- and C-termini,

Figure 3.7: Theoretical Diagram of an Immunoradiometric Assay (IRMA) or TSH in Man. (Courtesy of Dr G. Piatidis; see text for details.)

TSH I.R.M.A.

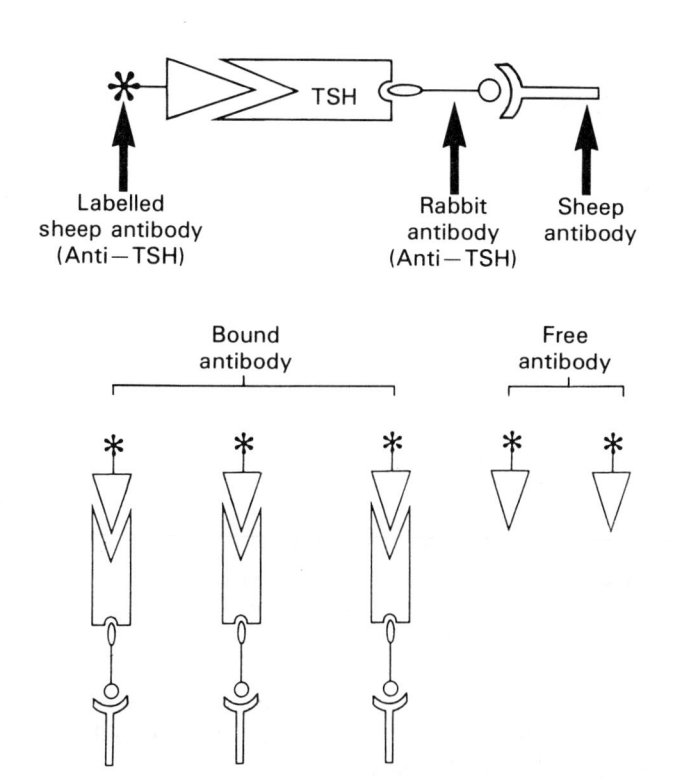

it is obvious that larger forms of ACTH will not be picked up. This becomes very important in patients with tumours that secrete these forms of 'big ACTH' (see Chapter 11). In such patients, ACTH levels by RIA may be extremely high, whereas values measured by IRMA may be low or undetectable. This discrepancy immediately suggests the presence of precursor forms of ACTH, a fact of some considerable clinical importance and previously only realisable following the time-consuming technique of chromatography (see below). It is likely that excess reagent assays will become increasingly popular in the coming years.

Chromatography

As the antibodies used in radioimmunoassay are usually directed principally towards one region of the molecule, there may be variation in other areas of the molecule which are not 'noticed' by RIA. For example, most RIAs designed to

28 Assays

detect and measure somatostatin 1–14 are in fact directed towards the common sequence of somatostatin 1–14 and pro-somatostatin, somatostatin 1–28. There is a substantial component of somatostatin 1–28 in the hypothalamus, and thus early studies on hypothalamic 'somatostatin 1–14' actually measured and reported on both forms. The fact that the RIA measures both molecular species was not originally realised, but is easily demonstrated if the components of somatostatin are separated according to their size and charge. This can be accomplished by chromatography, with the index sample being 'loaded' on to a gel column. Different molecular species elute off in different fractions, and the proportion of each species present can be determined by RIA of successive fractions. This is obviously a time-consuming operation, as 50 or more fractions from a single plasma sample may require assay. It is therefore not in routine clinical use, but is extensively used in investigational research. For example, it is now realised that many patients with the ectopic ACTH syndrome, and occasional patients with invasive forms of pituitary-dependent Cushing's syndrome, secrete forms of the ACTH precursor which are not normally present in the circulation. In acromegaly, GH may circulate in oligomeric forms consisting of two or more GH molecules combined: these may be detected by RIA but may not be biologically active, and thus treatment response in acromegaly may not be directly proportional to routine serum GH measurement. There is also evidence that prolactin may circulate in a variety of molecular forms, only some of which are biologically active. However, it is extremely important that the conditions of collection of samples for chromatography are carefully monitored to prevent artefactual aggregation or degradation. Thus, it was originally thought that the human pituitary secreted β-melanocyte stimulating hormone (β-MSH) into the circulation, and this was demonstrated chromatographically. Subsequent studies by Lowry and his colleagues conclusively showed that *fresh* acid extracts of samples only contained the large-molecular-weight precursor now known as β-LPH; with the passage of time after collection this was degraded to the smaller free β-MSH, which does not exist naturally in man.

More recently, even finer delineation of small differences in molecular structure have been possible using high pressure liquid chromatography (HPLC). This has produced such precise separation of molecular species that it may be combined with relatively crude means of actual detection, such as electrochemical detection.

Analysis of Data

As already indicated, the usual form for presenting data from a saturation analysis, as for bioassay, is as a dose-response curve. In this case the response, commonly the percentage of label that is antibody bound or the ratio of bound/free label, is plotted against the total hormone present in the tubes (dose) or log dose. A mathematical basis for the saturation analysis has been developed by a number of authors. There are certain differences in the individual approach, but common concerns are those of sensitivity and precision. Sensitivity is generally taken as the minimum quantity of substance detectable, and precision is an estimate of the assay reproducibility. If an assay is used routinely to determine hormone concentrations in clincal samples, the laboratory has to operate a system of quality control to ensure that the technique continuously produces highly reliable results. For the purposes of determining the variation of the quality of the assay, several 'control' tubes are run, including 'blanks' and samples from pools of known hormone content (generally 'low', 'normal' and 'high'). Laboratories aim for a between-batch variation of less than 15 per cent if using extraction and/or chromatography and RIA.

Routine Clinical Analysis

Establishing a saturation assay can be relatively time-consuming, but kits are available for the determination of certain hormones. Even with these a degree of expertise is required to obtain reproducible results. However, for clinical samples, a service should be available at the local or regional level in the UK. For more specialised or complex assays a supraregional assay service (SAS) was established in 1973, which makes reliable hormone and drug estimates available to chemical pathologists in all hospitals. These assays are expensive to perform, and care should be taken to ensure that requests for assays are clinically justified, and that the correct protocol is followed in obtaining samples. Most pituitary hormones are released in a pulsatile fashion and the rate of secretion is related to the sleep-wake cycle. It is therefore essential that samples are collected at the appropriate time of the day. Care should also be taken to ensure that patients are not receiving drugs that influence hormone release, and that they are not subjected to other stimuli affecting release. Many hormones are stress-released so that the patients should not be apprehensive (as might occur with repeated unsuccessful venepuncture). The secretion of several hormones (e.g. vasopressin) is dependent on posture.

Assays required for routine screening such as the gonadotrophins need a large throughput. This can be achieved in some instances by automation. In association with automation new methods of separating bound from free hormone have been developed, e.g. magnetic methods, and other forms of labelling have been developed e.g. enzymatic and fluorescent. Other assays such as those for ACTH and vasopressin requiring an extraction step inevitably have a slow throughput.

Radioimmunoassay will continue to dominate endocrinology over the next few years for many reasons, including its high sensitivity and the fact that multihead gamma counters allow the rapid processing of samples. Probably non-isotopic immunoassay will take over and eventually one might reach the state where all hormones are assayed by non-separation immunoassay techniques employing a non-isotopic label. By carrying out an assay entirely in the solid phase, it is even possible to envisage a rapid 'dip-stick' system for the estimation of the common peptide hormones.

Further Reading

Bangham, D.R. (1983) 'Assays and Standards', in C.H. Gray and V.H.T. James (eds), *Hormones in Blood*, 3rd edition, Vol. 5, pp. 256-99, Academic Press, New York

Butt, W.R. (1984) *Practical Immunoassay: the State of the Art*, Marcel Dekker, New York

Chard, T. (1982) *An Introduction to Radioimmunoassay and Related Techniques*, Elsevier Biomedical Press, Amsterdam

Chayen, J. and Bitensky, L. (1983) *Cytochemical Bioassays. Techniques and Clinical Applications*, Marcel Dekker, New York

Ekins, R.P. (1980) 'The Precision Profile; its Use in Radioimmunoassay Assessment and Design', *Ligand Quarterly*, 4, 33-44

Forsling, M.F. (1985) 'Measurement of Vasopressin in Body Fluids', in P.M. Baylis and P.L. Padfield (eds), *Posterior Pituitary*, pp. 161-92, Marcel Dekker Inc., New York

Gaddum, J.H. (1953) 'Bioassay and Mathematics', *Pharmacological Reviews*, 5, 87-134

Wood, W.G. and Sokolowski, G. (1981) *Radioimmunoassay in Theory and Practice*, Schnetztor-Verlag, Konstanz

4 THE HYPOTHALAMUS

Introduction

The hypothalamus sits at the gateway to the brain, monitoring electrical information from the limbic system and brain stem and transducing it *inter alia* into neurohumoral stimuli. Via the pituitary it controls many of the endocrine glandular elements of the body, and funnels electrochemical information regarding emotional and motivational processes into biochemical signals. As the principal non-neuronal 'output' system of the CNS it is obviously of primary significance, and its hormonal relationship with the pituitary will be dealt with in some detail. However, it also directly participates in many motivational behaviours, such as eating, drinking, and sexual behaviour, as well as certain vegetative functions such as temperature regulation. In addition it controls the sympathetic nervous system, of which it has been called the 'head ganglion'. Our increasing knowledge of neuropeptides and neuroamines suggests that the same substances controlling pituitary hormone release are also involved in behaviour modification, such that there appears to be an integrated system of endocrine and behavioural control. Thus, opioid peptides inhibit hypothalamic gonadotrophin releasing hormone (GnRH) release and therefore decrease circulating gonadotrophins, but they are also able to inhibit the sexual behaviour associated with changes induced by the central nervous system administration of the rat. Angiotensin II both stimulates vasopressin release from the neurohypophysis and increases the objective correlates of thirst. Food-seeking behaviour is also modified by a variety of neuromodulators, including dopamine, serotonin, cholecystokinin, GH-releasing hormone and bombesin. Although some work has proceeded in the direction of the localisation of such 'centres' within the hypothalamus, with a lateral hypothalamic 'appetite centre' and a medial 'satiety centre', it is now realised that most of these attempts at localisation are rather naive and somewhat premature. More complex networks are almost certainly involved, such as the suggested schema for the control of appetite shown in Figure 4.1. There is also considerable evidence for the hypothalamus as being the site of the biological 'clock(s)', which are responsible for the circardian (*circa dies* — 'about a day') or nyctohymeral (*nox, humor* — 'night-varying hormones') rhythms of hormone secretion and possibly behaviour. In this case, however, there is certainly good evidence in the rat that this resides in the suprachiasmatic nucleus. Overall, the hypothalamus and pituitary should be regarded as a dyad, the two poles — humoral and neural — serving in their own ways to preserve the stability of the *milieu intérieur* in the face of environmental and internal changes.

Historically, little was known of the hypothalamus until relatively recently. Although Forel outlined the area very beautifully within his 'regio subthalamica', the term 'hypothalamus' was only introduced by Wilhelm His in 1893. However,

Figure 4.1: Suggested Pathways and Peptides Involved in the Control of Appetite. (Redrawn after J.E. Morley.)

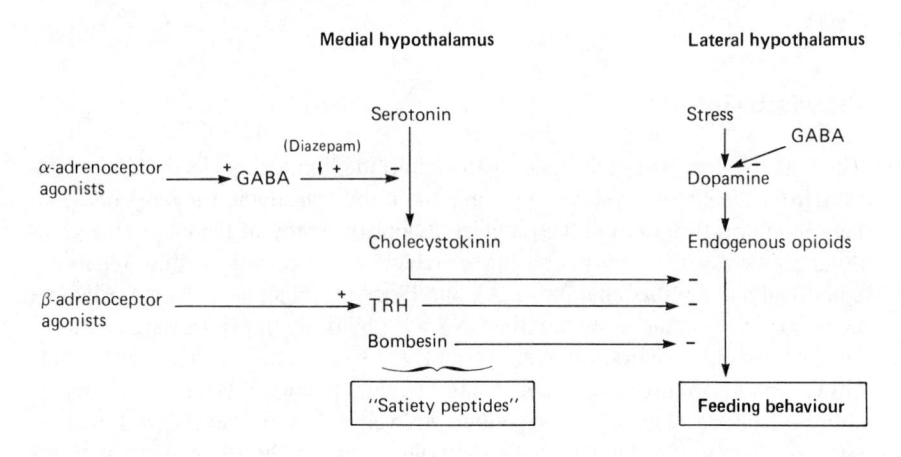

```
                    Medial hypothalamus              Lateral hypothalamus

                         Serotonin                       Stress
                 (Diazepam)                                 │        GABA
  α-adrenoceptor   +  ↓ +      —                         ↓ ←
  agonists    ────→ GABA ────→                         Dopamine
                                                          │
                                                          ↓
                        Cholecystokinin              Endogenous opioids
                         └──────┐                         │
  β-adrenoceptor      +         │    —                    │  —
  agonists    ──────────→ TRH ──┼──────────────────────── │
                                │                         │
                        Bombesin ──────────────────────── │ —
                            ⎵                             ↓
                    ┌──────────────────┐          ┌──────────────────┐
                    │ "Satiety peptides"│          │ Feeding behaviour│
                    └──────────────────┘          └──────────────────┘
```

its function was entirely unknown at this time. In 1881, Hermann Nothnagel had described the case of a man kicked by a horse, the man falling and hitting his head. The man then drank 3 litres of water and beer over a period of 3 h, with a gradual loss of his polydipsia over the next 4 days. Nothnagel believed that this traumatic polydipsia was caused by damage to the floor of the fourth ventricle. By the turn of the century the association of diabetes insipidus with pituitary damage came to be recognised. However, in 1920 a young houseman, Percival Bailey, was working for Harvey Cushing when he noted that he could produce polyuria in dogs by means of vascular damage to the hypothalamus while leaving the pituitary intact. Bailey and Bremer went on to show that the adiposogenital syndrome (what would now be known as hypothalamic obesity and hypogonadotrophic hypogonadism) was due to hypothalamic rather than pituitary damage — a finding that apparently 'infuriated' Harvey Cushing who believed in the primary importance of the pituitary.

Over the next twenty years or so the neurophysiologists researched extensively into subcortical structures, including the hypothalamus. Moruzzi and Magoun developed the concept of a diffuse 'reticular activating system', concerned with varying the level of arousal of the organism and acting independently of individual sensation, perception or cognition. Hess incorporated these ideas into a larger schema, in which the hypothalamus acted as a 'vegetative centre' for the sympathetic and parasympathetic nervous systems and produced integrated vegetative behaviour, i.e. behaviour orientated towards preserving the total body economy of the organism. For his work in this sphere he was awarded the Nobel prize in 1949. Meanwhile, the Scharrers and Wolfgang Bargmann were revealing the presence of neurosecretory granules in fibres running in the supraopticohypophysial tract. This tract, in fact, had been demonstrated by classic Golgi techniques in the rat as far back as 1894 by the Spanish neuroanatomist Ramon y Cajal, a flamboyant character who divided his time between the laboratory, where he carried out superbly detailed neuroanatomical studies, and the local bordello.

The final and definitive link between the glandular studies on the pituitary and neural studies on the hypothalamus was undoubtedly made by Geoffrey Harris. Fifty years ago he suggested that the hormones now known as TSH, ACTH, GH, LH, FSH and prolactin were ultimately controlled by the hypothalamus — and for good measure he included parathyroid hormone too. He developed the notion of the neurovascular link between hypothalamus and pituitary, and confirmed Wislocki and King's concept of portal blood flow being predominantly from hypothalamus to pituitary. This total *Gestalt* of hypothalamo-pituitary interaction was confirmed by the isolation, sequencing and synthesis of the hypothalamic releasing hormones, originally by Schally's and Guillemin's groups. As each new hormone has been described, year by year, the brilliance of Harris's original concept has been emphasised.

The Hypothalamic Hormones

Although Geoffrey Harris had accurately predicted the presence of hypothalamic hormones many years ago, it was not until the 1950s that the synthesis of hormones (oxytocin and vasopressin) in neurones of the hypothalamus was demonstrated, and only over the last 15 years that some of the hormones controlling the anterior pituitary have been isolated and synthesised. The hypothalamic regulatory hormones are usually present at very low concentrations in the hypothalamus such that their isolation has been particularly difficult. They are active in picogram or nanogram amounts such that 10 ng of releasing hormone may liberate 1 μg of trophic hormone. The first hormone to have its structure identified, *thyrotrophin releasing hormone (TRH)*, was found to be a tripeptide, the actual amino acid sequence being determined by synthesising the six possible combinations of amino acids and then modifying the N- and C-terminal residues and comparing the activities of the synthetic peptides with those of the native hormone. In addition to stimulating pituitary TSH release, TRH also releases prolactin. Indeed, it is possible that this latter function is the predominant effect of TRH *in vivo*. *Gonadotrophin releasing hormone (GnRH)*, a decapeptide, acts principally to stimulate the release of LH (hence it is also known as LHRH), and to a lesser extent FSH. Most endocrinologists consider that the relative proportions of LH and FSH released depend on the specific milieu, there being differential feedback of steroids and the peptide inhibin on each hormone, although there are still some who maintain that a separate FSH-RH is required to explain certain data. As TRH and GnRH are respectively three and ten peptide residues in length, it was considered likely that all the releasing hormones would be short polypeptides. This probably accounts for the delay in isolating *growth hormone releasing hormone (GHRH)*, recently demonstrated by two groups in carcinoid tumours from patients with acromegaly. Several forms of GHRH were identified with 37, 40 or 44 residues, respectively, and rat GHRH has been shown to contain 43 residues. However, the search for GHRH had led earlier to the discovery of a GH-inhibiting factor, a cyclic tetradecapeptide now known as *somatostatin*.

It was subsequently found that somatostatin had a wide range of inhibitory activities, including TSH, many gut peptides and even plasma renin.

Whereas corticotrophin releasing factor was one of the first of the hypothalamic hormones to be demonstrated by bioassay (by both Schally's and Guillemin's groups in 1955), it took a further quarter of a century to isolate the major peptide with ACTH-releasing activity — so-called *CRF-41*. This peptide is able to stimulate the release of all the pro-opiocortin peptides, both *in vitro* and *in vivo*, but it seems likely that other hypothalamic factors such as vasopressin and angiotensin synergise with CRF-41 to optimise ACTH secretion.

Although it had long been realised that *dopamine* was involved in the tonic inhibition of prolactin release, it took some time to accept that dopamine itself was secreted into the portal blood at a concentration sufficient to control lactotroph prolactin release. Other factors have been reported to modulate the lactotroph via the portal vein (including γ-aminobutyric acid (GABA), angiotensin, VIP and TRH), but dopamine retains its place as the major hormone in this process.

The labour necessary to isolate and identify these factors has been enormous, involving the extraction of up to half a million porcine or ovine hypothalami in some instances. This was acknowledged in the award of the Nobel Prize to A.V. Schally and R. Guillemin in 1979, although many other workers have been deeply involved, most recently W. Vale. It is sad that the original proponent of the concept of hypothalamic hormones, Geoffrey Harris, did not live to see his theories come to fruition.

Anatomy of the Hypothalamus

The hypothalamus is located in the ventral part of the diencephalon, where it forms the floor and inferior and lateral walls of the third ventricle. It extends from the lamina terminalis to a plane just caudal to the mamillary bodies.

It should be noted that the vast majority of work on the hypothalamus has been carried out in subhuman species, especially the rat. This species has fairly well-defined hypothalamic nuclei, and peptide and neuroamine pathways and localisation have been mapped in terms of rat cytoarchitecture terminology. In the human there is a much less clear differentiation into nuclear clusters, and cells in a given location (e.g. surrounding the third ventricle) may not be homologous to similarly sited cells in the rat. Most of the detailed localisation given below was obtained in the rat, so that possible differences in the human hypothalamus must be taken into account.

There are three major divisions of the hypothalamus (Table 4.1):

(1) The *nuclei which form the lower walls* of the third ventricles.
(2) The *tuber cinereum* and infundibulum, forming the anterior part of the floor of the ventricle. The median eminence forms a small 'blister' on the floor of the tuber cinereum, and is a much less significant structure than that seen in the rat.
(3) The *mamillary bodies* forming the posterior part of the floor of the ventricle.

Table 4.1: Principal Nuclei in the Human Hypothalamus. Part of the classification is based on rat material and many nuclei extend to more than one zone

Periventricular zone	Medial zone	Lateral zone
Suprachiasmatic	Medial preoptic	Lateral preoptic
Paraventricular	Ventromedial	Lateral hypothalamic
Arcuate	Dorsomedial	Mamillary
	Anterior hypothalamic	Tuberal
	Posterior hypothalamic	
	Premamillary	
	Supraoptic	

To these may be added:

(4) The *preoptic areas*. Although these are developed in the lamina terminalis, which is part of the telencephalon (forebrain), they are functionally related to the hypothalamus, especially with respect to the regulation of body temperature, sexual behaviour and TSH and growth hormone secretion.

Each of these divisions can be further subdivided into a number of nuclei. As has been emphasised already, these nuclei are not all distinct in human material, and it is difficult to establish which nuclei are homologous in the various subhuman forms (Figures 4.2 and 4.3). It is usually sufficient for the student to consider just those nuclei listed in Table 4.1. For the sake of convenience they have been grouped into those of the periventricular, the medial and lateral zones. The periventricular zone is that homogeneous area close to the ventricles, whereas the medial zone contains mostly clusters of neurones (i.e. nuclei with neuroendocrine activity), some of which control pituitary function. The lateral zone contains fibres connecting the limbic forebrain with the mesencephalon and some nuclei. Two types of nuclei may be seen, named on the basis of cell size, i.e. magnocellular and parvicellular. For example, the supraoptic and paraventricular nuclei are described as magnocellular and usually stand out in histological sections as areas of large, densely-stained neurones. The neurones which terminate directly on the capillaries of the portal vessels, the tuberoinfundibular neurones which produce the releasing hormones, are small and are described as parvicellular neurones they lie in a region also termed the hypophysiotropic area. Single specific functions cannot be ascribed to individual groups of hypothalamic nuclei nor may single specific functions be completely localised to an area, but there may be partial localisation of function for some peptides.

Localisation of Releasing Hormones

A great deal of effort has been put into the localisation of the hypothalamic releasing hormones. The earliest studies depended either on electrical stimulation, or on circumscribed lesions placed in nuclei or tracts believed responsible for the individual function. The major disadvantage of these techniques was that they also interrupted afferent pathways. More recently, specific areas from the hypothalamus have been dissected out and subjected to either bioassay or

36 *The Hypothalamus*

Figure 4.2: Magnetic Resonance Scan through a Midsagittal Section of Normal Human Brain. (Reproduced by kind permission of Dr J. Webb.)

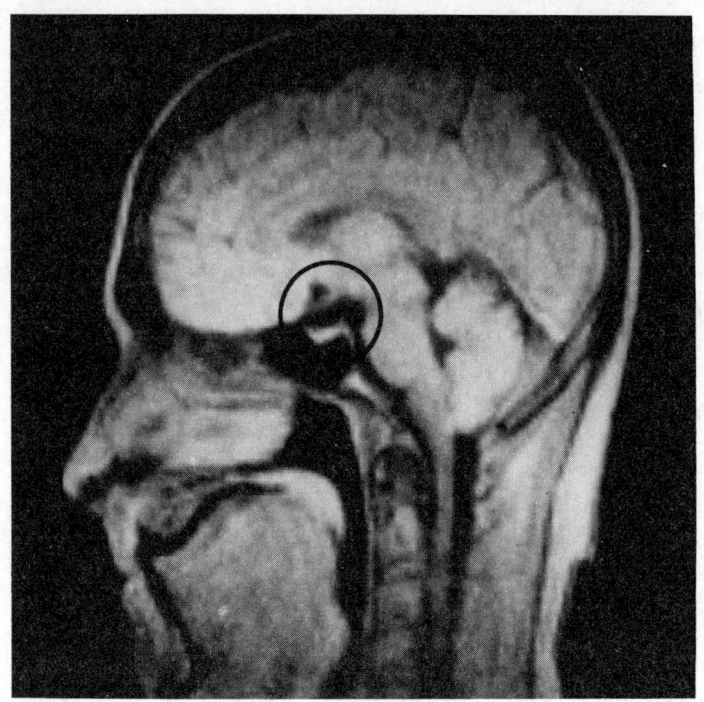

radioimmunoassay techniques to identify sites of production of specific hormones. Another powerful technique used to identify the location of the releasing hormones and neurohypophysial hormones is that of immunocytochemistry, using fluorescent or enzymic labels attached to specific antisera raised against the hormones (see Chapter 1).

It appears that the perikarya and axons of most neurones synthesising releasing hormones lie in a crescent-shaped zone on each side of the lower part of the ventricles in the rat (hypophysiotropic area) and extend into the medial basal hypothalamus. Much evidence is available concerning the location of the four releasing hormones whose structure is known. TRH occurs mainly in the dorsomedial nucleus, ventromedial nucleus and arcuate nucleus, but it is also found throughout the spinal cord. The localisation of LHRH is in two main areas, the arcuate nucleus and the preoptic area (especially the suprachiasmatic nucleus). There is considerable debate as to the respective roles played by these two areas in regulating gonadal function, and as to the extent to which they each release LHRH into the portal blood and hence control pituitary function. It appears likely that the arcuate nucleus is principally responsible for the tonic secretion of LHRH, whereas ovulation-related phasic increases may require augmentation by the preoptic area.

Figure 4.3: Principal Nuclei of the Human Hypothalamus. Nuclei: PV, paraventricular; PO, preoptic; A, anterior; DM, dorsomedial; P, posterior; SO, supraoptic; VM, ventromedial; A, arcuate; AP, adenohypophysis; N, neurohypophysis

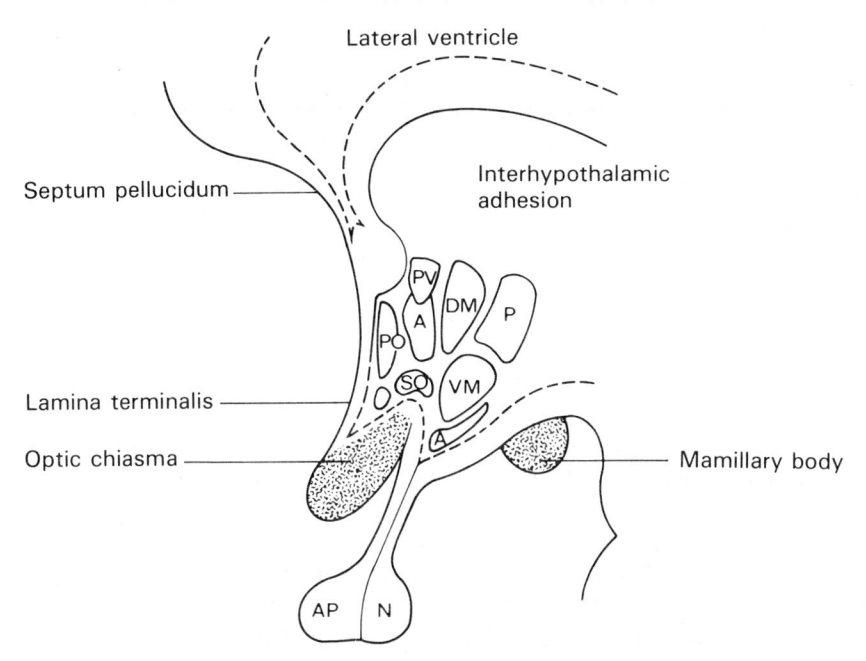

The principal ACTH-releasing peptide, CRF-41, is found mainly in the paraventricular nucleus, intermingled with cells producing vasopressin and oxytocin. There is also some evidence that some neurones in this complex may contain both CRF-41 and vasopressin, probably in the same synaptic vesicles.

The most recently identified releasing hormone, GHRH, was known from bioassay studies to be concentrated in the ventromedial nucleus in the rat. Studies in primates using GHRH antisera demonstrated some positive neurones in this nucleus, but surprisingly high concentrations of GHRH were also identified in the arcuate nucleus, and this is probably its major site of production.

Of the two release-inhibiting peptides, somatostatin is found in neurones located in the periventricular region which send axons along a tortuous course to terminate in the median eminence. The principal prolactin-inhibiting factor, dopamine, originates in neurones in the arcuate nucleus; these send processes to the median eminence in the so-called tubero-infundibular tract.

The sites of synthesis and storage of the neurohypophysial peptides vasopressin, oxytocin and neurophysin have been known for some time, and have been confirmed with immunocytochemical techniques. The hormones are mainly formed in the supraoptic and paraventricular nuclei, the supraoptic nucleus having the greater proportion of vasopressin-containing neurones. Recent evidence shows that vasopressin and oxytocin are also found in other areas, both inside and outside the hypothalamus.

38 The Hypothalamus

Figure 4.4: Main Afferent and Efferent Pathways of the Hypothalamus

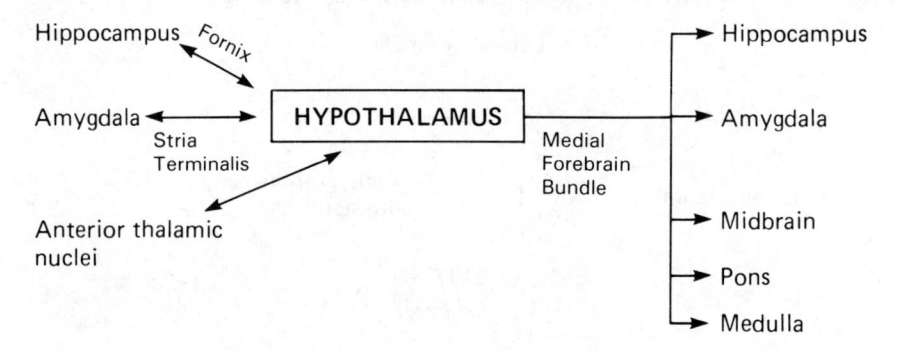

```
Hippocampus ←Fornix↘
                      ┌─────────────┐      → Hippocampus
Amygdala ←──────────→ │ HYPOTHALAMUS│ ─────→ Amygdala
           Stria      │             │ Medial
           Terminalis │             │ Forebrain
                    ↗ └─────────────┘ Bundle
Anterior thalamic                      → Midbrain
nuclei
                                       → Pons
                                       → Medulla
```

Connections of the Hypothalamus

Connections occur within the hypothalamus linking the various divisions (Figure 4.4), but they are difficult to study because of the extensive ascending and descending pathways entering the hypothalamus from other parts of the brain. The connections of the hypothalamus and extra-hypothalamic areas have been the subject of some study and may be summarised as follows (although this is a simplification of the present knowledge, which is still far from complete):

(1) *Afferent Connections*. These are principally from the *limbic system* and the *midbrain*.

(a) *Limbic areas:* the hypothalamus is part of the limbic system, which also includes the hippocampus, amygdala, and septal and habenular nuclei, as well as parts of the cortex (cingulate, orbitofrontal and pyriform). This system is evolutionarily 'old' as compared with the neocortex, and ablation and stimulation studies suggest that it is concerned with emotional/motivational behaviour and control. This is in contrast to the neocortex, which appears to be involved in perceptual and cognitive functions. Some workers have tried to sublocalise motivational function in the limbic system, for example the amygdala being conceived as controlling the 'significance' of emotive areas and the hippocampus being a 'motivational map' of significant objects. However, these attempts at classification are probably much too naive, although the present collaboration between neurophysiologists and behavioural scientists may well allow the attainment of the 'holy grail' of anatomical and behavioural correlation. For the present purposes it is sufficient to note that these limbic areas relay important inputs to the hypothalamus. One relay is found in the hippocampus and related areas (especially the septum) to the hypothalamus, the so-called fornix system, a second important relay is from the amygdala complex. The habenular nuclei also have efferents to the hypothalamus. It has been demonstrated that lesions or stimuli applied to each of these areas may have neuroendocrine correlates. Thus stimulation of the amygdala may increase LH and FSH, and iontophoretic morphine in this area may decrease LHRH release and inhibit ovulation. However it is still too early to delineate any specific role for limbic structures in neuroendocrine control.

(b) *Mesencephalon:* two important neuroamine projections run from the midbrain to the hypothalamus; one is a catecholamine noradrenergic input, principally from zones in or near the locus coeruleus running in the ventral noradrenergic bundle. The second projection is serotoninergic, consisting of 5HT-containing axons from neurones in the midline raphe nuclear system. Both projections ramify throughout the hypothalamus, but the 5HT system seems to have a particular tendency to terminate in the suprachiasmatic nucleus. Deafferentation studies have demonstrated that virtually all the noradrenaline and serotonin within the hypothalamus is derived from these inputs. By way of contrast, the high concentrations of hypothalamic dopamine are entirely intrahypothalamic within the tubero-infundibular system.

(c) *Cortical/retinal/thalamic:* there is some doubt as to whether the neocortex directly relays to the hypothalamus, although a pathway from the frontal cortex has been described. Afferents from the retina to the suprachiasmatic nucleus may be seen in some species, but, if present, they are probably polysynaptic. Most of the thalamic input appears to be via relays from mesencephalic cells.

(2) *Efferent connections.* The major output, in informational terms, is of hypothalamic releasing and inhibiting factors released into the portal system, plus the neurohypophysial hormones vasopressin and oxytocin released into the general circulation. The hypothalamus thus acts as a transducing organ, with complex electrical signals translated into changes in the amplitudes (and patterning) of chemical signals. These are in turn 'translated' and amplified in the pituitary, and pituitary hormones may stimulate their target organs with further signal amplification. There is therefore a cascade of events so that small perturbations in the CNS, e.g. in the limbic system, may, by progressive amplification and modification, produce significant modifications of the biochemistry and behaviour of the organism as a whole.

The hypothalamus also has efferent neural connections with the limbic system and midbrain. Direct relays are minimal to the medulla oblongata and non-existent to the spinal cord. However, polysynaptic chains of neurones enable the hypothalamus to exert a degree of control at both these sites.

The Medio-basal Hypothalamus

The medio-basal hypothalamus constitutes the final common pathway for neuroendocrine regulation, being the contact zone between the endings of the 'releasing factor' neurones and the capillaries of the hypophysial portal circulation. On the basis of both structure and function it has been divided into three zones.

(I) *The ependymal zone.* This inner layer lines the inferior part of the third ventricle. The large cuboidal ependymal cells send out elongated pinocytotic processes which pass through the median eminence to the portal capillary plexus.

These 'tanycyte' cells are believed to transport materials between the capillaries and the cerebral ventricles. It has been suggested that these ependymal cells recover 'hypothalamic' hormones or neurotransmitters from the CSF and deliver them to portal vessels, peptidergic neurones or pituitary cells. However, this remains to be decisively demonstrated as being of physiological importance.

(II) *The middle layer.* This layer contains the hypothalamo-hypophysial (releasing factor) neurones.

(III) *The palisade zone.* The palisade zone or external layer is the zone of connection between the axons of the tuberohypophysial tract (i.e. tuberoinfundibular neurones) and the capillary loops of the portal plexus. The structural arrangement is similar to that seen in the neurohypophysis. The endothelial cells of the portal capillaries are fenestrated. The vessel lumen is separated from the perivascular space by a basement membrane, and a second basal membrane separates the axonal endings from this space.

Neurotransmitter Regulation of Hypophysiotrophic Neurones

The neurosecretory cells are activated by neurotransmitters released at synaptic connections from the various afferent neurones converging on these cells. It is not clear whether all neurosecretory cells of a given type are triggered by the same neurotransmitter or neurotransmitters, or whether some are triggered by one and some by another. It might be that different neurotransmitters are involved in different responses — one set, for example, being involved in the stress response, and a second set in feedback responses.

Of the many putative transmitters present in the central nervous system, the ones most extensively studied in the context of the control of anterior pituitary function are acetylcholine, noradrenaline, dopamine and serotonin (5-hydroxytryptamine, 5HT). It has also been suggested that γ-aminobutyric acid (GABA) and glycine may play a role.

Clinical Aspects of Hypothalamic Disease

Hypothalamic function may be disturbed by infiltrative lesions of the hypothalamus, but more commonly by local lesions producing pressure and vascular disturbances, particularly of the portal blood supply. These disturbances may be classified into optic and functional deficits, the latter being subdivided into endocrine and non-endocrine. These deficits will first be reviewed, and then the possible causes will be examined in more detail.

Optic Deficits

A space-occupying lesion in the hypothalamus may expand inferiorly and thereby compress the optic chiasma from above. As the visual field on the retina is inverted and the optic nerve fibres retain their retinotopic patterning, the fibres first affected will be those representing the inferior portions of the temporal fields — a lower quadrantic bitemporal quadrantinopsia. However, it is uncommon for any lesion to be symmetrical, and a variety of field defects are seen in practice. Nevertheless, any chiasmal compression that is predominantly directed towards loss in the lower fields should raise the possibility of a primary hypothalamic defect.

Endocrine Deficits

A hypothalamic lesion that interferes with the releasing or inhibiting factors, or their access to the pituitary via the portal vessels, may cause changes in neuroendocrine function. As prolactin is under predominantly inhibitory control, changes in dopamine delivery to the lactotroph lead to hyperprolactinaemia. This is usually not marked and most hypothalamic tumours are associated with a serum prolactin below 1000 mU/litre; not infrequently, the serum prolactin is entirely normal (less than 360 mU/litre). Nevertheless, very occasionally in patients with hypothalamic lesions, serum prolactin may be considerably elevated to 4000–5000 mU/litre. Thus serum prolactin alone, in the presence of a mass lesion of the pituitary-hypothalamic axis, is only an approximate guide to the nature and location of the lesion. Progressive lesions will interfere with the synthesis or release of GnRH leading to a consequent decrease in the synthesis and release of pituitary gonadotrophins. In the early stages of such lesions the pituitary pool of LH and FSH will be maintained and their response to exogenous GnRH will remain normal. However, eventually the lack of endogenous GnRH stimulation will lead to a fall in the responsiveness of LH and FSH to the acute administration of GnRH, unless the patients are first primed (see below). This implies that poor gonadotrophin responses to LHRH may signify either a pituitary defect, or a longstanding lack of hypothalamic stimulation. The timing of the peak LH response to exogenous LHRH does not relate to the site of the lesion. Clomiphene is an anti-oestrogen and decreases the negative feedback effects of circulating oestrogens on LHRH release. Thus, in the clomiphene test (see Chapter 14), serum FSH and LH will rise in the normal subject. A normal gonadotrophin response to GnRH in the absence of a response to clomiphene generally indicates a hypothalamic defect in LHRH release or a disturbance of the portal system.

Growth hormone and ACTH are both stimulated by hypoglycaemia, which is assumed to produce hypothalamic stimulation of the release of GHRH and CRF. Severe acute exercise also releases GH and, to a lesser extent, ACTH, via hypothalamic pathways. The acute administration of the recently isolated releasing hormones GHRH and CRF-41 directly stimulates pituitary ACTH and GH release, although the peak ACTH response is slightly less than that seen in the presence of hypoglycaemia. The presence of a normal response to the releasing hormones and little or no response to hypoglycaemia suggests that the defect in hormone release occurs above the level of the pituitary cells themselves. Vasopressin has been used as a direct test of corticotroph function, but the test is unpleasant for the patient, not without danger, and there is also a probability that vasopressin has an additional suprapituitary site of action. Similarly, the arginine test for the GH reserve has the drawback of the lack of knowledge of the site at which arginine acts. Hypoglycaemia is usually induced by intravenous administration of insulin, 0.15 U/kg in adults or 0.10 U/kg in children, which produces a rapid response with glucose levels falling to less than 2.2 mmol/litre. This is equally rapidly reversed by the counter-regulatory hormones glucagon and adrenaline. In experienced hands the test is extremely useful and quite safe (see Chapter 14).

Defects in thyroid function are characterised by a fall in serum thyroxine. The absence of a compensatory rise in serum TSH suggests that the abnormality is (at least in part) above the level of the thyroid. The intravenous administration of TRH to normal subjects produces a rise in serum TSH at 20 min, with a partial return to basal levels by 60 min. If the TSH level is greater at 60 min than at 20 min, the 'delayed response', in the presence of a subnormal serum thyroxine, then usually the defect lies either in the release of TRH or in the access of the pituitary to TRH. It should be noted that the pituitary response to TRH may be apparently 'normal' in the presence of a subnormal thyroxine — it is the *inappropriate* relationship between the thyroid and TSH which indicates that there is pituitary hypothyroidism.

As the cells controlling vasopressin synthesis are situated within the hypothalamus, diabetes insipidus is frequently an early manifestation of hypothalamic disease. If the polyuria and polydipsia are severe, a single plasma sample of very high plasma osmolality in the presence of a low urinary osmolality is sufficient to make the diagnosis. More subtle changes which may need to be differentiated from psychogenic polydipsia and nephrogenic diabetes insipidus require a water deprivation test or a hypertonic saline infusion (see Chapter 14). There are no syndromes known, and hence no tests, for oxytocin deficiency.

Non-endocrine Deficits

As the hypothalamus controls a variety of motivational behaviour and vegetative regulatory functions, disease in this area may considerably upset these various functions. However, the disease must be widespread to produce clinical changes, and such disorders of hypothalamic function are surprisingly uncommon. When present, they usually include changes in food and water intake, sleep disturbances and disordered temperature regulation. Patients with a 'hypothalamic syndrome' may exhibit marked hyperphagia, and may often become extremely obese. Patients with the Prader-Willi syndrome, a congenital disorder of unknown aetiology, probably have hypothalamic obesity and tend to die at a relatively young age of obesity-induced hypoventilation — the Pickwickian syndrome. It is associated with mental retardation and defects in the hypothalamo-pituitary-gonadal axis. Changes in thirst, either polydipsia or adipsia, may also be seen in hypothalamic disorders. The coexistence of diabetes insipidus and a decrease in thirst sensation is particularly dangerous as the patient may become severely dehydrated. The sleep disturbance which may become manifest is continual somnolence, or diurnal drowsiness with nocturnal insomnia. Such patients may therefore wander nocturnally, sometimes in search of food. Poor temperature regulation is often not realised at an early stage, and these patients may become comatose on general wards, either if the wards are badly heated in the winter, or if the patients are allowed to sunbathe in the summer.

Hypothalamic Disorders

Craniopharyngiomas. These comprise tumours derived from remnants of Rathke's cleft and are usually (but not always) suprasellar in location. Although most commonly seen in childhood and young adults, they may present at any age. Pathologically the tumours have a mixed histological picture but always contain elements of stratified squamous epithelium and often some degree of keratinisation. Cysts are characteristic, often multiple, and typically contain a yellowish fluid. These cystic tumours may enlarge to compress the optic chiasma and cause varying degrees of endocrine deficit, usually including diabetes insipidus. In childhood, failure of growth or delay in entering puberty is usually seen. In addition, compression of the aqueduct of Sylvius may produce the typical symptoms and signs of raised intracranial pressure, namely headache, vomiting and papilloedema. Long-standing optic-tract compression may lead to optic atrophy. These tumours are very often calcified, so that they may be diagnosed from plain skull radiology by the flecks of suprasellar calcification and often the backward 'splaying' of the dorsum sellae. The spread of the tumour can be outlined by CT scanning, but in the absence of calcification a normal CT scan does not necessarily exclude the presence of a craniopharyngioma. Endocrine defects are variable and the serum prolactin may be normal (especially in childhood). Surgical biopsy is usually necessary for diagnosis and the surgeon may proceed to clearance of the tumour. The tumours are moderately radiosensitive, and most authorities advise postoperative radiotherapy to eradicate all tumour remnants and prevent recurrence. Some surgeons feel that radiotherapy is not indicated where removal is said to be complete, but it is difficult to be entirely sure that this is the case. Even with radiotherapy the recurrence rate is 10–20 per cent, although the tumours are relatively slow-growing. There is evidence that radiotherapy together with decompressive surgery is as effective as radical attempts at total excision, and the former has a lower mortality and morbidity; treatment of recurrent tumour by radiotherapy is certainly superior to reoperation. Endocrine replacement therapy may be required subsequently. A recent survey has indicated that at least part of the previously high mortality of this disease in childhood results from the fact that patients with electrolyte disturbances (cortisol and vasopressin deficiency) may receive inadequate treatment during times of stress (febrile illness, gastrointestinal upset, surgical procedures, etc.). Shunting of the cysts may be necessary acutely to lower raised intracranial pressure, and aspiration through a burr hole may alleviate symptoms and can be repeated on several occasions.

Occasionally craniopharyngiomas may be entirely intrasellar. An epidermoid cyst may represent a variant of the craniopharyngioma.

Histiocytosis X. This rare condition subsumes three syndromes, having in common the presence of tumorous masses of foamy histiocytes. In 'eosinophilic granuloma of bone' these masses are unifocally located in a long bone which may undergo pathological fracture. Letterer-Siwe disease is a rampant manifestation of the disorder in which widespread dissemination of histiocytes throughout soft tissues, including bone marrow, occurs over a short period of time; it is usually a disorder of childhood, and in most cases is rapidly lethal. Hand-Schuller-Christian disease is of intermediate morbidity, with scattered clumps of these histiocytes appearing at different sites and most typically in the region of the hypothalamus and in the bones of the skull vault. Endocrine defects are variable, but usually include diabetes insipidus, and proptosis may occur. Radiotherapy may be attempted to shrink the lesion, but it is not always effective.

Germinomas. Germinomas are seen in the region of the pineal and anterior hypothalamus, and constitute the majority of the so-called 'pinealomas'. True tumours of the pineal cells are very rare. Germinomas may present in a similar way to craniopharyngiomas (visual loss, diabetes insipidus, hypopituitarism) and are also preferentially seen in children and young adults. There is a male predominance in those that arise in the pineal area. However, due to their location they may also present with signs of pressure on the optic tegmentum, including one or more signs of Payrinaud's syndrome (convergent nystagmus, Argyll-Robertson pupils and failure of upgaze). In addition, patients with pineal germinomas may present with isosexual precocious puberty, although this is an uncommon cause of this syndrome. This interesting phenomenon may be due to the tumour compressing the inhibitory (?pineal) pathways controlling LHRH release, but may also be due to true tumour secretion of human chorionic gonadotrophin (hCG), as is seen in patients with testicular germinomas. This may cause an apparent rise in serum LH due to cross-reaction in the assay. Occasionally hCG is found in the CSF, even when it is apparently absent from the serum. The presence of hCG in the circulation of a (non-pregnant) patient with a hypothalamic tumour is virtually diagnostic of a pineal germinoma or a teratoma with chorionic elements. Radiotherapy is the treatment of choice as these tumours are supremely radiosensitive and may disappear entirely with treatment. Surgical removal is too hazardous in most patients, but a small biopsy may be attempted. Alternatively the response of a suspicious mass to radiotherapy may be used, as failure to shrink substantially suggests that the tumour is not a germinoma. As the tumour may seed down into the cord in 10 per cent of cases, many authorities consider that prophylactic radiation of the spinal cord should be given, although in childhood this will unfortunately limit truncal growth. Long-term prognosis following full craniospinal irradiation is still uncertain, but apparent cure in the short term is usually seen. Chemotherapy has not so far been particularly successful. Overall survival rates are similar to craniopharyngiomas, being of the order of 60–75 per cent.

Chordomas. Chordomas are rare tumours arising from the primitive notochord, either distally (in the region of the sacrum) or proximally extending from the clivus to the suprasellar region. They are histologically quite distinctive, containing lobulated cords of frothy-looking ('physaliferous') cells, but may present like pituitary tumours with suprasellar extensions. Although slow-growing, they are highly invasive locally. Surgical removal can be difficult, and since the tumours are relatively radio-resistant, the eventual outcome of treatment is poor. However, they are not incompatible with reasonable long-term survival, and a recent survey demonstrated occasional survivors at up to 10 years.

Hamartomas. These benign mixtures of tissue that resemble cerebral grey matter may be an incidental radiological or post-mortem finding. Occasionally they may be associated with deficiencies of some or all of the hypothalamic releasing hormones. They may also be seen in patients with isosexual precocious puberty, and in one noted case immunostaining of the hamartoma demonstrated GnRH neurones. Presumably in this case there was a functional disconnection between the LHRH cells and the normal inhibitory inputs from the rest of the hypothalamus. In the absence of visual pathway disturbance or other compressive problems, it is probably judicious to avoid biopsy and merely observe with high-resolution CT scans at regular intervals. Hamartomas of the hypothalamus may also secrete CRF or GnRH, and be clinically associated with Cushing's disease or acromegaly.

Tuberculomas. Tuberculomas may appear *de novo* as a hypothalamic mass lesion, probably in a patient predisposed to tuberculosis (e.g. Asian immigrants in the UK) or as a long-term sequela of tuberculous meningitis. Diagnosis is by biopsy unless there is clear evidence of tuberculous disease by CSF analysis. Failure of response to antituberculous chemotherapy demands surgical intervention.

Neurosarcoidosis. It is important to realise that sarcoidosis may present neurologically without any evidence of systemic sarcoidosis. Sarcoid granulomas may invade the pituitary and/or hypothalamus and give rise to a spectrum of defects in this region. There is a suggestion that neurosarcoidosis is particularly common in West Indians. Analysis of the CSF usually demonstrates a mild monocytosis together with an increased protein content, which may be so high as to increase greatly the CSF viscosity. The granuloma should be revealed on CT scanning, but tissue diagnosis (not necessarily from the hypothalamic granuloma) should be obtained. Other neurological manifestations of neurosarcoidosis are usually present and treatment with immunosuppressants such as corticosteroids may lead to dramatic shrinkage of the mass. However, the long-term prognosis is not favourable.

Arachnoid Cysts. Cysts lined by a thin layer of arachnoid and containing clear CSF have been reported throughout the CNS. In the hypothalamic area they may present as raised intracranial pressure and/or endocrine changes, the symptoms being relieved by aspiration of the cyst cavity. It is thought that some cases of the empty sella syndrome arise from an arachnoid cyst that has been 'pinched off' from arachnoid herniating into the stalk. The suprasellar cysts are clearly visible on CT scanning as dense black areas that do not usually enhance with contrast medium. Refilling of the cyst after aspiration may be a problem, in which case marsupialisation of the cavity is necessary.

Isolated Defects of Hypothalamic Releasing Factors. These may be congenital or acquired, and it is increasingly being realised that many previously considered abnormalities of pituitary hormone secretion are secondary to changes of the releasing factors. These include isolated GH deficiency causing short stature, isolated gonadotrophin deficiency (Kallman's syndrome) and isolated ACTH deficiency. In many cases they are associated with other 'midline' abnormalities. They will be described in the appropriate chapters on each pituitary hormone.

Further Reading

Banna, M. (1976) 'Craniopharyngioma: Based on 160 cases', *British Journal of Radiology, 49*, 206-33
Elde, R. (1979) 'Localisation of Hypophysiotrophic Peptides and Other Biologically Active Peptides within the Brain', *Annual Review of Physiology, 41*, 587-602
Magnen, J.L. (1983) 'Body Energy Balance and Food Intake: a Neuroendocrine Regulatory Mechanism', *Physiological Reviews, 63*, 315-73
Meites, J. and Sonntag, W.E. (1981) 'Hypothalamic Hypophysiotropic Hormones and Neurotransmitter Regulation; Current Views', *Annual Review of Pharmacology, 21*, 295-322
Mills, R.P. (1984) 'Chordomas of the Skull Base', *Journal of the Royal Society of Medicine, 77*, 10-16
Tixier Vidal, A. and Gourdji, D. (1981) 'Mechanism of Action of Synthetic Peptides on Anterior Pituitary Cells', *Physiological Reviews, 61*, 974-1011
Williams, P.L. and Warwick, W.E. (1981) 'The Hypothalamus', in *Gray's Anatomy*, 36th edition, pp. 965-74, Churchill Livingstone, Edinburgh

5 CONTROL OF HORMONE SECRETION

When the importance of the anterior pituitary in controlling the endocrine system became apparent in the 1960s, it was named the conductor of the 'endocrine orchestra'. As indicated in the previous chapter, it now seems that the pituitary is the leader of the orchestra and it is the hypothalamus that is the conductor. When the pituitary was believed to be the site of hormone control, it was postulated that anterior pituitary hormone concentrations were maintained by negative feedback control from target organs. This system is still believed to be important in the control of anterior pituitary hormone production, but additionally it is now known that nervous control via the hypothalamus is at least equally significant. Realisation of the possible link between the central nervous system and the endocrine system came longer ago than one might imagine. In 1818, first Gill and later, in 1935, Vimont reported that unilateral castration caused atrophy of the contralateral hemisphere of the cerebellum in an experimental animal. A few years later, Berthold, in his experiments on testicular transplants, implicated the nervous system as a target organ, and in 1856 Maetre de San Juan described gonadal hypoplasia in men with agenesis of the olfactory lobes. This observation was subsequently confirmed by many groups of workers, but this and much subsequent work, which was in essence the beginning of 'neuroendocrinology', was ignored by mainstream biologists.

The realisation of the existence of neurotransmitters and neuromodulators was also important in the development of neuroendocrinology. In 1877 Reymond had suggested a chemical transmission from motor neurones to striated muscle. A rather surprising and early insight into this aspect came from Schiefferdecker, who in 1905 put forward the theory that endocrine substances could be secreted by neurones as a means of communication either between neurones or between a neurone and an effector cell, either a muscle or a gland. This theory was based both on his own observations and on Tigerstedt's autonomic irritability theory, which postulated that irritation or stimulation is caused by metabolic products of internal secretion. The first neurotransmitter to be investigated in detail was acetylcholine; the opening chapters of this story appeared in 1914 when Dale published his paper on the action of certain esters and ethers of choline in which the nicotinic and muscarinic actions of acetyl choline were distinguished. In the same year Elliot wrote of the possibility of chemical transmission in the autonomic nervous system. Adrenergic transmission was recognised when, in 1931, Cannon and Bacq described sympathin, a hormone produced by sympathetic action on smooth muscle. These many strands eventually came together and in 1936 Marshall described the process whereby in higher animals the internal rhythm is related to external phenomena, partly 'through the central nervous system and probably through the hypothalamus upon the anterior pituitary and thence upon the testis and ovary'. Another important strand was the development of control theories. Weiner suggested that the concept of feedback mechanisms and cybernetics could be applied to biological systems, and in 1949 Hoskins introduced these ideas into the area of endocrinology.

General Concepts of Biological Control Systems

Once the science of cybernetics was established, it became potentially easier to understand the workings of the nervous and endocrine systems, the two principle control systems of the body. In the nineteenth century there were a number of prophets of the science of control systems, including Maxwell, who in 1864 had expounded on the importance of machines (such as those of James Watt) in a paper entitled 'The theory of governors'. However, it was not until around 50 years ago that the science of machines was truly established. Its birth was heralded by the publishing of a relatively little-known book by Jacques Lafitte, *Reflexions sur la science des machines*. It is now recognised that self-regulating machines are servo-mechanisms, the abbreviation 'servo' being derived from the Latin for 'slave'. Central to the science is the concept of control, a special relationship between two machines or parts of machines so that one part regulates another. The essential point is that the source of energy is dissociated from the source of instructions. The control signal only requires a very small amount of power, so there is amplification of the controlling signal. It is not sufficient to understand individually diverse forms of control; it is necessary to combine these relations if one is going to grasp the essentials of the organism as a whole. There is a need to study the pattern of interconnections, the network of relations. Important in understanding this network is the principle of meshes or closed circuits (also termed loops), a concept first introduced in 1847 by Kirchhoff in his paper on electrical networks. Such loops are fundamental in the schema of servo-mechanisms and it is from them that reflex and reactive structures are formed. All goal-directed organisation demands closed circuits with their inherent feedback loops. Such a system is essential for the maintenance of the *milieu intérieur* as proposed by Claude Bernard in 1878.

Thus there are a number of basic characteristics of a control system. First there must be a sensor or error detector sensitive to the variable being regulated, and which changes its signal rate as the variable changes. Then there must be a continuous flow of information from the sensor to an integrating centre. This afferent pathway can be nervous or humoral. The integrating centre generally receives information from many receptors, each possibly responding to different types of stimuli. The output or command signal from the centre is therefore the result of integration of many and often conflicting items of information. The command signal travels via the efferent pathway, again nervous or humoral, to the effector organ. Finally, the ultimate effects of the change in output by the system must be made known (fed back) to the sensor initiating the events. The type of feedback normally seen in biological systems is negative feedback, a system in which an increase in the output ultimately results in a decrease in that output.

This obviously leads to stability and is crucial to the operation of homeostatic mechanisms. Where there is a complete circuit, sensor-controller-effector-sensor, the term 'closed loop' is applied; if an external agent acts on the system, the term 'open loop' is applied. As well as negative feedback, there are also positive feedback loops in which the initial disturbance in the system initiates a series of events which amplify the disturbance. Such a system leading to explosive events is clearly unstable so that it can only be tolerated where there is an obvious end-point. Examples of positive feedback may be found in neuroendocrine systems, as for example in the release of oxytocin during labour. Oxytocin, released as a result of stimulation of cervical receptors, causes increased uterine activity so that the infant is pushed further into the birth canal; this in turn produces additional stimulation of the cervical receptors. Positive feedback also operates to produce the surge of gonadotrophins at ovulation. Normally steroids (mainly oestrogen) feed back negatively on gonadotrophin release, but when a critical concentration is maintained for a period of time, positive feedback occurs and induces greatly augmented release of LH and FSH. Unstable positive feedback loops are also seen frequently in pathological situations when minor perturbations are continually amplified and the system breaks down.

In engineering terms the simplest system is an on/off system, which depends on the effector being turned on or off by a sensing device. Such a system inevitably has oscillations. More complex systems are required to provide a constant output of the controlled variable. Proportional control systems adjust the output in proportion to the degree of fluctuation in the controlled variable. The simple proportional system will still have minor errors that can be corrected by an integral control system in which the rate of change of the output is proportional to the input. Such a system may be used as the basis for understanding physiological control mechanisms. Regulatory systems are far more complicated than any of these systems, as the physiological set points can be varied according to diurnal cycles, metabolic states, etc. As already mentioned, there are many separate sources of input, and physiological regulation often depends on simultaneous excitatory and inhibitory outputs. However, the basic concepts can be readily applied to most neuroendocrine control systems.

Some reflex arcs of a control system seem to lack a receptor and an efferent pathway. This is typified by the simple negative feedback system which is believed to operate in the control of the secretion of anterior pituitary hormones. For example, TSH is released from the anterior pituitary into the systemic circulation and subsequently acts on the thyroid gland to stimulate release and synthesis of thyroid hormones. The circulating concentration of thyroid hormones then feeds back at the level of the pituitary gland, thus providing a means of controlling the circulating level of thyroid hormones. In this example the change in TSH secretion may be seen as the efferent pathway, the thyroid as the effector organ, but there appears at first sight to be no receptor or afferent pathway. In fact it appears that the pituitary gland itself is sensitive to the circulating concentration of free thyroid hormone. Feedback of the hormone at the level of the pituitary is termed 'long-loop' feedback, as the source of thyroxine is spatially distant from

50 Control of Hormone Secretion

Figure 5.1: Typical Control Loop for Pituitary Hormone Release. Some pituitary hormones do not have target gland feedback (e.g. prolactin). Not all pathways have been proved for every hormone

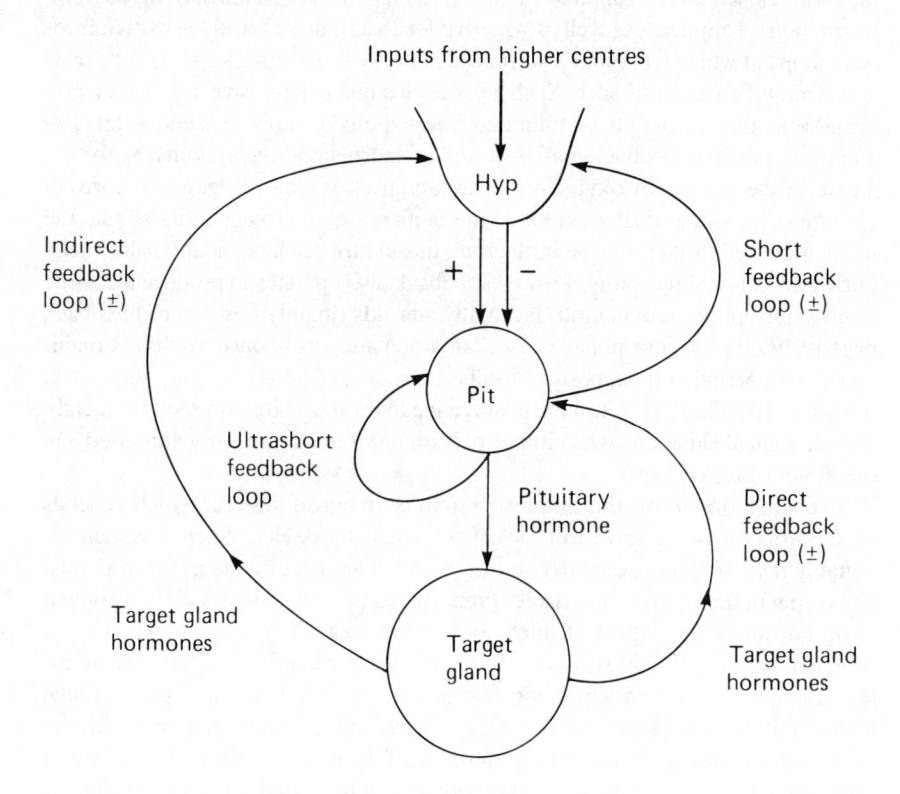

the pituitary (Figure 5.1).

The control of the posterior pituitary is rather different from that of the anterior pituitary. As the secretory cells of the neurohypophysial system are themselves neurones, the secretory process is rather more akin to that for hypothalamic releasing factors than for anterior pituitary hormones. However, feedback systems still operate in the control of vasopressin secretion. For example, an increase in the osmotic pressure stimulates the osmoreceptors, which results in increased vasopressin release. The hormone is transported by the plasma to the kidney, where it promotes reabsorption of water so that the plasma osmolality falls. Similarly, if the systemic blood pressure drops, vasopressin is released causing water retention, which in the long term can aid in the maintenance of blood pressure. In the short term, vasopressin also acts to produce vasoconstriction which contributes to the return of blood pressure to normal values. It may also be related to drinking behaviour, so that homeostasis is obtained through several effector mechanisms.

Action of Hypothalamic Controlling Factors

In terms of the secretion of anterior pituitary hormones, superimposed on the simple negative feedback system is control from the hypothalamus. Feedback may also operate at the level of the hypothalamus. Thus there is evidence that corticosteroid released from the adrenal cortex (by the action of ACTH) feeds back, not only at the pituitary to influence ACTH release directly, but also at the hypothalamus to influence CRF release. Furthermore, pituitary hormone secretion may also modulate hypothalamic hormones: thus an increase in serum prolactin will lead to an increase in the release of hypothalamic dopamine (short-loop feedback). Similarly, growth hormone increases hypothalamic somatostatin secretion and thus inhibits its own release. *Direct* effects of pituitary and hypothalamic hormones on their own release (ultrashort-loop feedback) have also been described. The nature of the releasing factors has already been discussed in Chapter 2. Although releasing hormones have been named in terms of one single anterior pituitary hormone whose secretion they control, the hypothesis of one hypothalamic hormone, one pituitary hormone is now known to be false. One hypothalamic hormone can modulate several pituitary hormones (e.g. TRH on TSH and prolactin) and a given pituitary hormone can be affected by various hypothalamic factors (e.g. TSH by TRH and somatostatin).

In addition to the feedback system, release of hypothalamic peptides is influenced by inputs from higher centres relaying information from external and internal stimuli and by 'biological clocks'. As with any other neurone, whether a hypothalamic neurosecretory neurone fires depends on the total sum of inhibitory and stimulatory impulses impinging on it — either the 'ayes' or the 'noes' have it. The exteroceptive organs, the ears, eyes and skin, etc., as well as the interoceptive senses all send impulses either directly or via other regions to the hypothalamic secretory neurones. Other influences such as local steroid hormone concentrations may additionally influence the release and cyclical rhythmicity. Temporal organisation is characteristic of a multiplicity of biological functions. Some rhythms are generally believed to be manifestations of self-sustained oscillators or biological clocks. In the context of a biological clock, the suprachiasmatic nucleus appears to play an important part, at least in the rat. In man there seem to be two classes of circadian oscillators. The first, the sleep-wakefulness cycle, is relatively labile and so can deviate fairly readily from a 24-hour rhythm. The second class, which includes hormone secretion as well as the rhythms of body temperature, urine excretion, cell division, enzyme synthesis and numerous other functions, has a strong power for self-conservation. Studies in blind subjects have shown that certain hormonal rhythms entrained to the sleep-wakefulness cycle can be shifted from this and can cycle independently. Indeed, ACTH may be more strongly entrained to light-dark than sleep *per se*. All known mammalian circadian rhythms are entrained by the light-dark cycle, and evidence in experimental animals indicates that this is a result of interaction between light, the pineal and the supra-chiasmatic nucleus. In the human it must be assumed that factors other than light-dark cycles are important as entraining agents of circadian rhythm;

for example, social cues and knowledge of time would be expected to have a strong influence. Light, however, does appear to influence circadian rhythms in the human, as it has been reported that blind subjects are not as precisely synchronised to a 24-hour day as sighted subjects, and their approximately 25-hour 'day' may represent a return to a more primitive rhythm.

Those hormones that show particular variation over the 24-hour span are ACTH, cortisol, GH, prolactin and to some extent the gonadotrophin and TSH. There is considerable speculation as to the physiological significance of the various patterns. Since GH, prolactin and LH during puberty are largely secreted during sleep, it has been suggested that sleep is an important mechanism for synchronising the metabolic and tissue changes that occur during puberty. The spontaneous adrenocortical activation in the early morning has been postulated as preparatory for everyday motor activity. Nevertheless, each hormone appears to have its own distant rhythmicity. Thus TSH increases from mid-morning to peak at about 23.00 h, irrespective of sleep, and prolactin peaks in the early morning hours. Serum growth hormone pulses at about 2- or 3-hourly intervals throughout the day, and much longer pulses occur at night, strictly entrained to 'slow wave' or non-dreaming sleep. By contrast, ACTH increases in secretion throughout the night to reach highest levels at 07.00–08.00. Plasma renin activity dips during dreaming sleep (REM sleep) and plasma noradrenaline rises with REM sleep.

Whereas night work allows growth hormone to continue pulsing during the non-dreaming sleep during daytime, it takes 7 to 10 days for the ACTH rhythm to become entrained to the new activity pattern. It may be that some of the behavioural problems associated with shift work can be ascribed to the inertia of this system in responding to changes. It is evident that the 'week on-week off' night duty worked by some nurses, for example, requires continuous modulation of ACTH rhythms. Similar considerations apply to the temporal changes associated with rapid travel between East and West, i.e. so-called 'jet lag'. These time relationships can also have a significant bearing on the effects of treatment, for example corticosteroid therapy. Typically these steroids are given without significant reference to biological rhythms, and in long-term treatment the benefit derived may be accompanied by undesirable side-effects.

Abnormal patterns of cortisol secretion are seen in Cushing's syndrome and in patients with psychotic depression. Interestingly, in contrast to normal subjects, in patients with aldosteronism caused by adrenal disease ACTH or a related peptide may control circadian rhythms of aldosterone. An abnormal circadian pattern of GH secretion is also seen in acromegalics and of prolactin in patients with hyperprolactinaemia. Thus it is possible that knowledge of the normal 24-hour secretory pattern of hormones and the possible variations can provide a diagnostic tool as well as allowing a mechanistic insight into many clinical syndromes.

Mechanism of Action of Hypothalamic Peptides on Anterior Pituitary Cells

The mechanism by which the hypothalamic hormones affect pituitary secretion has not been fully determined, but the availability of synthetic hypothalamic peptides has allowed a number of studies to be carried out. *In vitro* studies have indicated that hypothalamic peptides exert a dual effect on the secretion of adenohypophysial hormones — a rapid transient action on hormone release and a long-term action on hormone synthesis. The mechanisms involved in hypothalamic hormone action are clearly dependent on the organisation of the target cells. In common with other protein-secreting cells of the endocrine system, those of the anterior pituitary contain a large store of membrane-bound granules. The hormones, or rather their large precursor forms, are synthesised on membrane-bound polysomes where translation of specific RNA occurs. As messenger RNA has to be a minimum of 200 to 250 bases long in order to maintain attachment of the ribosome to the endoplasmic reticulum, in general, smaller peptides are produced as fragments released from larger prohormones. In addition there is a 'leader' sequence that is removed as the prohormone is secreted into the endoplasmic space from the pre-prohormone. Sometimes the prohormone contains multiple copies of single peptides, and in other structures the remaining fragments are functionally 'cryptic' (i.e. no known function at present). In the case of the ACTH precursor pro-opiocortin, some of the co-secreted products appear to have functions independent of ACTH. The prohormones are discharged into the lumen of the rough endoplasmic reticulum and are transported to the smooth reticulum of the Golgi zone where secretory granules form. During that transit the secretory product undergoes several chemical transformations, such as addition of sugars and sulphated components. The newly formed granules are stored in the cytoplasm before being discharged via exocytosis. An intracellular mechanism called crinophagy allows degradation of excess secretory granules. Observations suggest that hypothalamic neurones release hormone from this preformed store. Regarding synthesis, the exact action of the hypothalamic hormones is not clear. For example, LHRH has been variously reported to preferentially stimulate incorporation of glucosamine (suggesting acceleration of glycosylation) or proline into LH. The possibility has not been ruled out that an additional site of action could be reduction in the degradation of anterior pituitary hormones. This is good evidence that the hypothalamic hormones act at the outer membrane. A preparation of TRH bound to a high-molecular-weight dextran has been shown to be effective, and radioactive TRH has been shown to bind to membrane fractions or intact pituitary cells with an affinity constant similar to that observed for the biological activity of the native hormone. However, there is also evidence for internalisation of TRH and GnRH.

Despite extensive studies the involvement of cyclic AMP or cyclic GMP has not been unequivocally demonstrated, and although calcium has been implicated, its contribution is not clear. Nevertheless, cyclic AMP is strongly suspected as being the second messenger in the response to GHRH and is at least partly involved in the actions of somatostatin and LHRH (GnRH). There is also recent evidence suggesting that the dopaminergic inhibition of prolactin release occurs with a fall in cyclic AMP at the so-called D_2 receptor site. Recent studies have centred on the involvement of microtubules and microfilaments.

Neurotransmitters in the Release of Anterior Pituitary Hormones

In addition to feedback effects, the tuberohypophysial neurones are acted on by classical neurotransmitters. Monoaminergic and cholinergic pathways are important. Dopamine, serotonin and noradrenaline pathways are the principal control systems, but adrenergic and histaminergic neural control systems are also found. Dopaminergic neurones involved in the regulation of the anterior pituitary arise mainly in the arcuate nucleus of the hypothalamus and are distributed to the median eminence. Other dopaminergic systems include the nigrostrial pathway, which arises in the substantia nigra and distributes to the caudate nucleus and other forebrain structures, and the mesolimbic system, which projects to the cortical limbic nuclei. The cell bodies of the noradrenergic pathways all lie outside the hypothalamus. The majority of the adrenergic fibres involved in neuroendocrine control arise from areas adjacent to the locus coeruleus in the brain stem and from cells close to the nucleus of the vagus nerve. These fibres ascend to terminate in many brain regions, with a particularly important input to the hypothalamus. There is also a less prominent adrenergic pathway. Most of the serotoninergic neurones supplying the hypothalamus also arise in the brain stem (raphe nuclei). In addition there may be an intrinsic serotonin pathway within the hypothalamus analogous to the tuberohypophysial dopamine pathway.

Cholinergic neurones appear to be associated with all the defined nuclei in the hypothalamus. Also demonstrated in fairly high concentrations in the hypothalamus and median eminence is GABA. Neuropeptides found in nerve endings in the hypothalamus include substance P, met-enkephalin, β-endorphin, angiotensin II, neurotensin, gastrin, cholecystokinin, VIP and dynorphin.

Despite extensive studies extending back over more than a decade, there is remarkably little agreement as to the functional importance of these putative regulators. In many cases a number of studies demonstrating, for example, that serotonin stimulates the release of LHRH may be matched by others showing no effect, or even inhibition. Part of the explanation for these discrepancies lies in the use of agonist or antagonist drugs of uncertain specificity, or of amine precursors whose subsequent metabolism is ill-defined. No drug can be considered to be entirely specific, but certain inconsistencies seem to epitomise the approach of using drugs 'of which we know little in an organism of which we know less'. Furthermore, very often the neuroendocrine response to pharmacological manipulation is dependent uopn the given situation, such as the state of the oestrous cycle for LHRH, pubertal development for GHRH and the corticosteroid milieu for CRF. Other approaches, such as the local application of putative neurotransmitters into the CSF or on to the hypothalamus directly, or the use of hypothalamic fragments or cultures *in vitro*, must also take into account the tremendous disruption of neuronal circuitry that these techniques involve. Systemic administration of drugs must also allow for the rate of absorption and metabolism, and, most importantly, whether the drug penetrates the 'blood-brain barrier'. This constraint is based on the observation that many molecules do not appear to have access to parts of the CNS, suggesting a selective barrier to entry in these areas. This 'barrier' may be very highly selective, with very small changes in molecular geometry greatly influencing accessibility. Overall it is usually only *relatively* impermeable depending on the concentration of the drug and the duration of its effect. A further level of complexity comes from the fact that certain parts of the brain are functionally outside the barrier; these include the area postrema of the medulla (including the 'vomiting centre'), many circumventricular nuclei, and the pituitary and median eminence. Studies have also employed antisera, and similar considerations apply in these instances. Systemic administration of drugs is usually the only means of investigating neurotransmitter control of endocrine function in man, so despite these provisos this approach is frequently employed. However, the judicial use of a variety of agents together with appropriate comparisons with data derived from the rat do allow certain tentative statements to be made.

Prolactin

There is extensive data suggesting that dopamine is the major prolactin-inhibiting factor (PIF) acting directly on the pituitary lactotrophs to inhibit prolactin release. This is true both in normal man and in most patients with prolactinomas, and is the basis of the therapeutic usefulness of bromocriptine. Additionally GABA inhibits prolactin release at a pituitary level, but is about two orders of magnitude less effective than dopamine; it appears to be an important PIF in birds, but its role in mammals remains uncertain. Within the hypothalamus, there is evidence that GABA may *decrease* dopamine release and thus indirectly *increase* serum prolactin. It is also reasonably well established that 5HT stimulates prolactin secretion, most probably through activating a prolactin-releasing factor (PRF — see below). There are few publications suggesting important roles for acetylcholine or noradrenaline in the control of prolactin release, but recent work indicates stimulation by histamine and inhibition via histamine-2-receptors.

TRH provides a powerful stimulus for prolactin release and thus prolactin concentrations may change as TRH is stimulated or inhibited. Recent studies have also demonstrated that vasoactive intestinal polypeptide (VIP), which is present in the hypothalamus, can directly stimulate the lactotrophs, but the control of VIP itself remains to be elucidated. Endogenous opioid peptides (enkephalins, endorphins and dynorphins) clearly stimulate prolactin release in rat and man, with the bulk of evidence demonstrating that this occurs via disinhibition of the dopaminergic tubero-infundibular pathway. However, there is little evidence that this opioid control of prolactin is important in man. Finally, angiotensin seems to stimulate the lactotrophs to release prolactin, whereas DKP, a cyclic degradation product of TRH, directly inhibits prolactin release by the lactotroph.

Growth Hormone

In most species, probably including man, there is good evidence for noradrenergic stimulation of growth hormone release, probably through α_1-receptors. More detailed studies have suggested that these are principally of the α_2 subclass, as α_2-agonists and antagonists (such as clonidine and yohimbine, respectively) appear to be most active. It is uncertain as to whether these receptors are pre- or postsynaptic and whether they act through GHRH or somatostatin. Activation of β-adrenoceptors appears to inhibit GH release by increasing somatostatin. Both acetylcholine and 5HT stimulate the secretion of GH and there is a suggestion in man that a muscarinic cholinergic link is a final common pathway for many stimuli of growth hormone secretion, but excluding the rise in GH induced by hypoglycaemia. Histamine appears to stimulate growth hormone release through histamine-1 receptors. GABA also increases serum growth hormone. Evidence with regard to dopamine is confusing. This is partly because dopamine itself does not penetrate the blood-brain barrier. In addition the dopamine precursor L-dopa is also metabolised to noradrenaline and the effect of dopamine appears to depend on the pre-existing level of serum growth hormone. One interpretation of the data is that dopamine exerts a dual control on GH release. There is convincing evidence that dopamine stimulates somatostatin release and hence lowers GH. Under some circumstances dopamine may directly inhibit pituitary GH release, and it seems possible that dopamine also stimulates GHRH release. At low plasma concentrations, GH secretion would be stimulated by the release of GHRH, and in the presence of already elevated levels of GHRH and GH, the inhibitory role of dopamine becomes manifest. The suppression of serum GH by dopamine or dopamine agonists in some patients with acromegaly is due to the presence of dopamine receptors on the somatotrophs.

The neuropeptide control of both somatostatin and GHRH is poorly understood, but opiates clearly stimulate GH secretion, probably via changes in GHRH. Under certain circumstances TRH can also stimulate growth hormone release. Certain of these controlling pathways are shown in Figure 5.2.

TSH

The hormone TSH is controlled by hypothalamic TRH, for which there is good data in favour of an excitatory noradrenergic input. This pathway may be involved in the release of TRH and TSH in response to cold stress. Dopamine inhibits TSH release and there is evidence that, under certain circumstances, noradrenaline and dopamine directly modulate TSH release at the level of the thyrotroph. Inhibition appears to be the predominant effect of 5HT on TRH.

In the rat opiates are powerful inhibitors of TRH release whereas in man slight stimulation is seen. There is little evidence in man that any of these control mechanisms are important, but the neonatal surge in TSH secretion may be noradrenergically mediated.

Figure 5.2: Some of the Main Factors Causing an Increase (+) or Decrease (−) in Growth Hormone Release

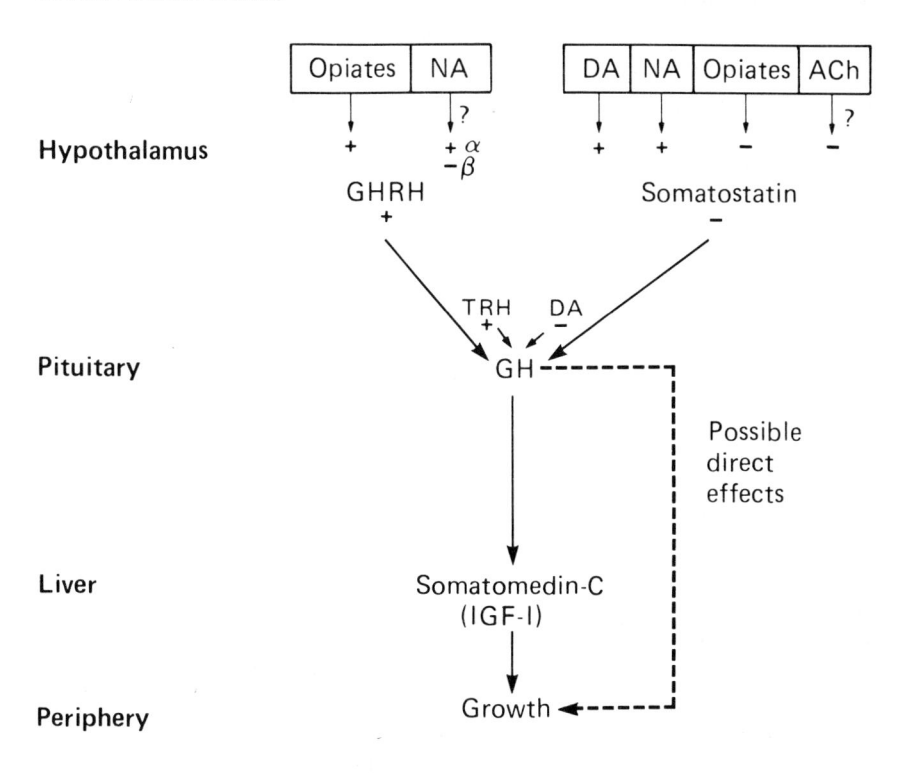

```
                    ┌─────────┬────┐      ┌────┬────┬─────────┬─────┐
                    │ Opiates │ NA │      │ DA │ NA │ Opiates │ ACh │
                    └────┬────┴─┬──┘      └─┬──┴─┬──┴────┬────┴──┬──┘
                         │      │ ?         │    │       │       │ ?
Hypothalamus             +      + α         +    +       −       −
                                −β
                        GHRH                    Somatostatin
                          +                          
                             \       TRH   DA       /
                              \       +     −      /
Pituitary                      →     GH ←         ←--------┐
                                      │                    │
                                      │                    │ Possible
                                      │                    │ direct
                                      │                    │ effects
                                      ▼                    │
Liver                           Somatomedin-C              │
                                   (IGF-I)                 │
                                      │                    │
                                      ▼                    │
Periphery                          Growth ←----------------┘
```

ACTH

Early work by Ganong and his colleagues in the rat purported to show that noradrenaline was involved in the suppression of CRF release, and many subsequent studies supported this theory. However, there is an increasing minority opinion that noradrenaline is principally excitatory to ACTH release. The very limited data in man are certainly more in accord with this latter view. These effects via CRF must clearly be distinguished from direct effects of catecholamines on the pituitary corticotrophs. In the rat there is a functional pars intermedia and this appears to have a direct innervation leading to β-adrenoceptor stimulation (and dopamine inhibition) of the release of ACTH and related peptides. By contrast, the non-innervated corticotrophs of the pars distalis are not generally responsive to applied catecholamines except possibly at high pharmacological concentrations. The scanty data in man (who does not have a functional pars intermedia) suggest that endogenous noradrenaline stimulates the release of CRF at α-receptors whereas dopamine has little or no influence. Acetylcholine, serotonin and histamine probably all stimulate ACTH release in rat and man. One hypothesis suggests that the stress-induced release of ACTH is mediated via the mesencephalic noradrenergic projection, whereas the circadian rhythm of ACTH is contingent upon a serotoninergic input from the suprachiasmatic nucleus. This is an attractive theory, but it requires further experimental support.

Opiate alkaloids and opioid peptides have varying effects on ACTH in the rat, but uniformly suppress ACTH release in man, possibly via the noradrenergic pathway.

Feedback of steroids, principally corticosterone in the rat and cortisol in man, occurs at both hypothalamic and pituitary levels, as already indicated.

Gonadotrophins

There is considerable data to indicate that there is a noradrenergic excitatory input to GnRH secretion in the rat, and this input is especially important in mediating the ovulation-associated augmentation of LHRH output. It has been suggested that an increase in this noradrenergic input is responsible for the gradual rise in GnRH output during pubertal maturation, and an opioid inhibition of this linkage can modulate changes in GnRH associated with ovulation. According to some workers the major input of noradrenaline is in fact through its metabolite, adrenaline. The role of acetylcholine is unclear whereas serotonin has the capacity to suppress GnRH tonically, but to facilitate its ovulation-related release. More controversial is the role of dopamine, for which there is a vast corpus of research demonstrating both stimulatory and inhibitory functions. McCann has suggested that there are two dopaminergic inputs to GnRH release at two separate anatomical sites. Of the peptides there is some work indicating the involvement of VIP in GnRH release. As mentioned earlier, much effort has been put into elucidating the role of endogenous opioids which are powerful suppressors of the hypothalamo-pituitary-gonadal axis.

In the human there is no clear evidence for the involvement of any of the neuroamines in GnRH release. The work of Knobil and his colleagues indicates that an *invariant* hypothalamic signal is quite sufficient to allow normal sexual function in the male primate and normal menstrual function in the female primate. It thus appears that the primate has relatively little dependence on neuronal influences, and steroid feedback (both positive and negative) at the pituitary level can alone maintain a monthly cyclicity. Nevertheless, there is good evidence that opioid inhibition (at a hypothalamic level) modulates GnRH pulsatility throughout the menstrual cycle, and is almost certainly responsible in part for the inhibition of LHRH release seen in some patients with hypothalamic and hyperprolactinaemic amenorrhoea. Furthermore, recent work has demonstrated that preovulatory rises in LH tend to occur between 03.00 and 05.00, indicating entrainment to a neuronal clock.

In seasonal-breeding animals the pineal has antigonadotrophic effects, and during non-breeding seasons pineal influences produce gonadal quiescence through inhibition of LHRH release. It is uncertain whether this is mediated by melatonin, another metabolite of 5HT, or possibly by a pineal peptide. The role of the pineal in man remains uncertain, although there is some disputed evidence for a fall in pineal activity occurring at the time of puberty.

Vasopressin and Oxytocin

As with the anterior pituitary hormones, there is considerable debate regarding the neuroamine and neuropeptide control of vasopressin and oxytocin. However, it appears reasonably well confirmed that cholinergic pathways are important in the control of vasopressin secretion. Muscarinic receptors may be important, although they appear to terminate on the magnocellular neurones. The nicotinic receptors are in close proximity to these cells. It is currently impossible to make a clear comment on the central role of catecholamines in vasopressin release. Noradrenaline has been found to be both stimulatory and inhibitory. The tuberoinfundibular dopamine system appears to decrease vasopressin secretion, but the response to opiates is complex. For example, relatively large doses of morphine administered into the third ventricle of the rat produce stimulation of vasopressin release followed by inhibition, whereas low doses produce only inhibition. Opiates directly inhibit the release of both vasopressin and oxytocin at the neurohypophysial level. In addition, it is postulated that there is an opiate regulation of dopamine release such that increased opioid activity decreases dopamine release and hence leads to a rise in vasopressin. Although the use of mixed agonists-antagonists in man has been said to reveal a stimulatory role for endogenous opioids, in normal circumstances the effect of applied opiates is inhibitory and this may be useful in the syndrome of inappropriate secretion of vasopressin.

Clinical Considerations

The principal relevance of our knowledge of neurotransmitter function in neuroendocrinology relates to the effects of drugs on pituitary hormone secretion. Thus, the fact that dopamine is the dominant inhibitor of prolactin release suggests that dopamine antagonists will lead to hyperprolactinaemia. This is in fact found and is particularly important in the case of the major tranquillisers and the antiemetics metoclopramide and domperidone. Similarly, dopaminomimetic agents such as bromocriptine are important drugs in the treatment of elevated serum prolactin levels, whatever the cause. Dopaminergic agents are also clinically useful in the treatment of growth hormone-secreting tumours, and in patients without pituitary tumours L-dopa has been used as a stimulus to test growth hormone reserve. However, it is evident that our lack of knowledge of the mechanism of this effect rather limits the clinical usefulness of the test. Adrenergic or noradrenergic drugs also have some clinical import, in that clonidine is a more widely used test than L-dopa for the testing of growth hormone reserve in children and young adults. It is known that this occurs through α_2-adrenoceptors, but clear stimulation of growth hormone release in normal subjects is only seen in childhood or during puberty. There is also a poor correlation between clonidine testing and the results obtained with the more conventional insulin-induced hypoglycaemia. Amphetamine increases central catecholamine activity and this is probably responsible for the rise in ACTH and cortisol seen with this drug in acute studies. It will also be recalled that serotonin stimulates ACTH release, probably via CRF. It has been shown that patients with pituitary-dependent Cushing's syndrome occasionally respond to the serotonin antagonist cyproheptadine with a fall in ACTH and clinical improvement. However, cyproheptadine has a variety of pharmacological actions and it has also been demonstrated directly to suppress ACTH release from pituitary cells *in vitro*. This suggests that it may interfere with the process of hormone exocytosis *per se*, possibly by influencing the calcium mediator calmodulin, and this may be unrelated to any interaction with serotonin receptors.

Although the histamine$_2$-receptor antagonist cimetidine can elevate serum prolactin if given parenterally in high doses, there is no evidence that oral therapy with either cimetidine or ranitidine will cause hyperprolactinaemia.

Agents that increase GABA neurotransmission, such as the anticonvulsant sodium valproate, have been said to lead to lower plasma ACTH in patients with Nelson's syndrome and in some patients with Cushing's syndrome. However, the evidence is not clear cut and the conclusions are controversial at present.

Of the neuropeptides, the hypothalamic hormones themselves are dealt with in other chapters. Opioid peptides increase serum prolactin and growth hormone while suppressing ACTH, LH and vasopressin. It is possible that the opiate alkaloids butorphanol or oxilorphan could be useful in suppressing vasopressin release in patients with the syndrome of inappropriate ADH secretion (SIADH, Schwartz-Bartter syndrome), but this has not been formally tested. Similarly the opiate antagonist naloxone increases ACTH, LH and FSH in normal subjects and markedly increases the gonadotrophins in certain women with amenorrhoea, but this has yet to be applied clinically. No other neuropeptides have been investigated from the point of view of their clinical usefulness.

In terms of normal physiology we are again lacking information. Although the process of pubertal maturation in the rat appears to involve both adrenergic and opioid pathways, this does not appear to be the case in man. Similarly, although it is tempting to speculate that pituitary tumours in man might arise secondarily to hypothalamic releasing hormone and/or neurotransmitter dysfunction, there is no substantial evidence to support these notions. By the time they present clinically, such tumours are relatively autonomous of hypothalamic control. Subtle changes in neuroendocrine function are certainly seen in some neuropsychiatric syndromes (Parkinson's disease, Huntington's chorea, depressive illness, mania), but the variability of the phenomenon does not suggest that there is a common disorder in neurotransmitter function. Further studies are required to define whether these changes are a response to the disordered mental state rather than a reflection of a common neuropathological process.

More detailed knowledge of hypothalamo-pituitary control mechanisms has also increased our ability to localise pathological lesions, although the tests in use are not as precise as had previously been hoped. Thus many patients with 'hypopituitarism' and absent cortisol and growth hormone responses to hypoglycaemia show a response to the respective releasing hormones CRF and GHRH, suggesting that the defect is hypothalamic in origin. However, the 'delayed' TSH response to TRH is not always seen with hypothalamic tumours, and poor gonadotrophin responses to LHRH do not locate the level of the pathological process. In addition, few of the suggested prolactin stimulation or inhibition tests are definitive in demonstrating the presence or absence of small pituitary tumours. Nevertheless, no endocrine test can be properly interpreted in the absence of a good knowledge of the underlying control mechanisms, and it seems likely that our increasing knowledge of such mechanisms will improve the validity and reliability of neuroendocrine test procedures.

Further Reading

Krieger, D.T. (1979) *Endocrine Rhythms*, Raven Press, New York

McCann, S.M. (1982) 'The Role of Brain Peptides in the Control of Anterior Pituitary Hormone Secretion', in E.E. Muller and R.M. Macleod (eds), *Neuroendocrine Perspectives 1*, pp. 1-22, Elsevier Biomedical Press, Amsterdam

Meites, J. (1980) 'Interactions between Hypothalamic Neurotransmitters and Pituitary Function (Symposium)', *Federation Proceedings, 39*, 2888-94

Reichlin, S. (1982) 'Neuroendocrinology of Pituitary Regulation', in J.A. Givens (ed.), *Hormone-secreting Pituitary Tumours*, pp. 27-44, Year Book Medical Publishers, Chicago

Rusak, B. and Zucker, I. (1979) 'Neural Regulation of Circadian Rhythms', *Physiological Reviews, 59*, 449-520

Turek, F.W., Swan, J. and Earnest, D.J. (1984) 'Role of the Circadian System in Reproductive Phenomena', *Recent Progress in Hormone Research, 40*, 143-83

6 MECHANISMS OF PEPTIDE HORMONE ACTION

Introduction

Hormones act as stimulators or modulators of reactions in specific cells by altering enzyme activity. Thus they play an important role in homeostasis, influencing both the concentration of circulating nutrients and the rate at which they are used, as, for example, in the maintenance of plasma glucose, or the control of salt and water balance. They also have a morphogenic action, being important in growth, maturation and ageing. In addition, some hormones may influence the nervous system and its responsiveness to particular stimuli. Yet other hormones may be described as 'permissive'. This means that their presence is essential for the action of other hormones but thereafter they have no modifying effect. A physiological example is the release of glucose from glycogen (as shown in Figure 6.1) in which the effect of adrenaline on glucose release depends on the permissive presence of cortisol.

Although hormones circulate throughout the body and reach every tissue, they only produce their effects on certain organs — the so-called target organs. The peptide hormones can produce a wide variety of responses in many tissues, but it now appears that the primary events are essentially similar for most hormones.

The action of a peptide hormone on its target organ is due to its interaction with specific receptor sites, usually located in the plasma membrane. Receptor binding or recognition is followed by a number of steps, namely transduction of the signal, transmission, reception, modulation of the response and its termination. Transduction entails the mobilisation of a second messenger, generally cyclic AMP or calcium, which initiates the intracellular response. Until recently, most peptide hormones have been thought to act via cyclic AMP, although there is increasing evidence that calcium may also be important. However, cyclic AMP does not seem to be involved in the response to hormones such as growth hormone, prolactin and insulin. In such cases enhanced protein synthesis and/or changes in membrane permeability appear to be involved. In these instances it has been suggested that activation of a membrane protease liberates a peptide regulator, or that an intrinsic receptor kinase is activated leading to phosphorylation of a membrane constituent.

In common with other areas of cell biology, great strides have been made in our understanding of the mechanisms underlying receptor-related events. Considerable advances have been made from the turn of the century (when the receptor concept was first proposed). Now, the protein oligomers responsible for ligand recognition have been identified; the membrane-located reactions subsequent to ligand binding have been elucidated; and awareness has developed of the importance of hormone receptors as the potential site of disordered function in disease. The concept of specific receptors dates back to the first decade of the century,

Figure 6.1: Action of Cyclic AMP in the Breakdown of Glycogen

```
                          Adrenaline
                              │
                              ▼
                 Activated adenylate cyclase
                              ╲  ATP
    Signal             Cyclic AMP
      │                       │
      │                       ▼
      │           Activated cyclic AMP –
      │           dependent protein kinase
      │                       │
      │                       ▼
      │              Activated phosphorylase
      │                     kinase
      │                       │
      ▼                       ▼
  Amplification        Phosphorylase b → a
   of signal                  │
      │                       ▼
      ▼
    Effect         Glycogen ─────────→  Glycogen
                (n glucose units)      (n-1 glucose units)
```

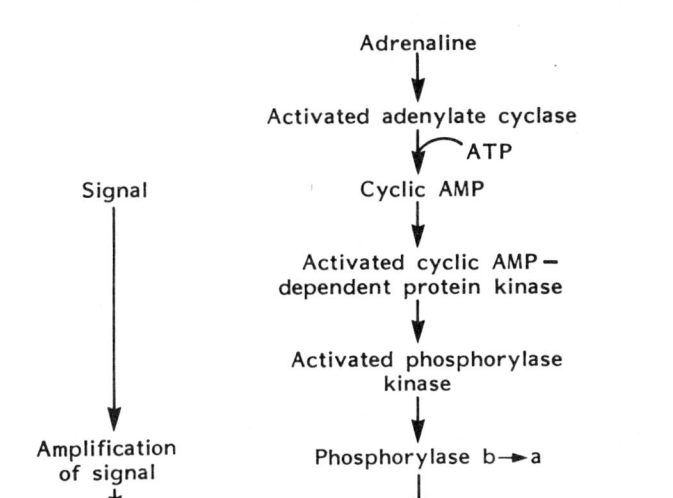

when Langley recognised that cells contained a 'receptive substance' which affected the 'chief substance' concerned in the production of contraction or secretion, and with which neuromuscular drugs and internal secretions probably reacted. A short time later, Ehrlich, as a result of his interest in antibody specificity, postulated that highly specific side chains are present in the cell protoplasm which could serve as receptors with which chemotherapeutic drugs could combine. The recognition by Gaddum that receptor occupancy determines the magnitude of the pharmacological response has been the basis of quantitative analyses of the action of ligands with receptors. Subsequent landmarks were the hypothesis of 'spare receptors' for hormones and drugs, and the recognition that there are subclasses of receptors, such as the renal and vascular receptors for vasopressin. More recently, the original picture of a fixed receptor structure has been modified so that the receptors are envisaged as subject to conformational changes on activation.

Since the receptors for peptide hormones lie on the outer cell membrane, there has to be a method of transferring the signal to the inner cell contents; considerable attention has centred on these so-called 'second messengers'. In examining the mechanisms involved in adrenaline-induced increases in hepatic phosphorylase, Sutherland and Roll discovered cyclic AMP, a discovery which was to revolutionise ideas on the biochemical mechanisms of hormone action. They found that adrenaline and glucagon stimulated the formation of a heat-stable factor from plasma membrane fractions which increased the activity of phosphorylase kinase. This enzyme catalyses the phosphorylation of inactive phosphorylase to the active form. The heat-stable factor was identified as cyclic AMP, and the enzyme responsible for its production was named adenylate cyclase. Some 10 years later it was shown that cyclic AMP produces its effects by controlling a single class of intracellular enzymes, the protein kinases. For many years attention has centred on cyclic AMP as the second messenger, but more recently interest has returned to calcium. In 1947 it was shown that calcium administration could induce muscle contraction at the site of injection and over the next five years evidence accumulated to show that calcium played a central role in excitation-stimulus coupling. It was later also shown to be important in stimulus-response coupling. Recognition of its role in hormone actions came much later.

Hormone Receptors

The steroid hormones, thyroid hormones and vitamin D do not act through the mediation of cyclic AMP, but through an entirely different mechanism. These groups of hormones may be considered together as they have relatively similar actions entailing the activation of cytosolic or membrane receptors leading to the regulation of nuclear transcription with altered (generally increased) production of messenger RNA. In the case of steroids, the hormone crosses the cell membrane and binds to a high-affinity cytoplasmic receptor. These receptors are found in two forms. The binding of steroid hormones with the larger form (with a high sedimentation constant of 8S) results in conversion to the 4S complex. Translocation of this complex to the nucleus results in conversion to a complex with a sedimentation rate of 5S, which binds to chromatin. This in turn leads to changes in the activity of nuclear-DNA-dependent RNA polymerase, and hence to changes in the rate of production of messenger RNA. In the case of thyroid hormones, there is an active transport mechanism for them in the cell membrane. As with steroid hormones, there is a cytoplasmic binding protein, but the mechanism of entry of thyroid hormones into the nucleus is different from that of steroid hormones. However, once in the nucleus, the DNA-dependent RNA polymerase is again stimulated, translating RNA from a DNA template.

Recently there has been considerable progress in the isolation and analysis of cell membrane receptors. Most of the recognition molecules characterised appear to be large oligomeric proteins with molecular weights in the range 100 000 to 30 000, so that only a relatively small portion of the receptor would appear to be embedded in the membrane. The receptor represents no more than 0.01 per cent of the plasma-membrane protein, there being 5000 to 10 000 receptors per cell. The insulin receptor has an immunoglobulin-like structure, comprising two pairs of polypeptide chains (α and β) linked by disulphide bridges to form a four-chain oligomer, so that more than one binding site is available. The receptor for somatomedin C (Chapter 8) has been found to have a similar subunit composition, as have the subunits for GH, TSH and LHRH.

Receptor mobility appears to be necessary for hormone action. This concept was developed by Cuatrecasas and his colleagues. In 1975, they postulated that, after hormone binding, the receptor underwent a conformational change which allowed it to bind to or influence other membrane proteins, thus initiating the response. This conformational change is a highly specific receptor response to

Figure 6.2: Postulated Changes in Hormone Receptors Following Hormone Binding

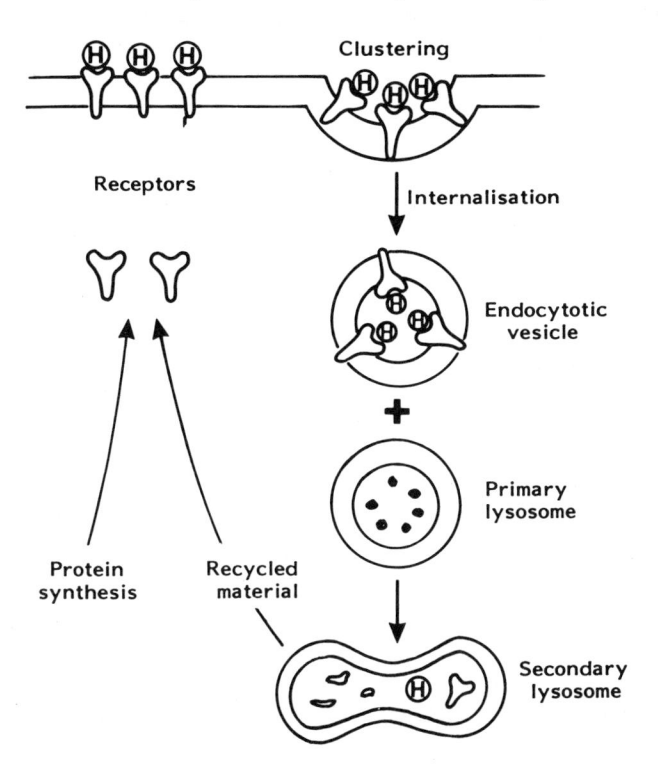

interaction with the ligand. However, other reactions, such as binding of the receptor to antibodies that cross-link receptors, can also lead to receptor activation and thus stimulation of the cellular response. A number of receptor antibodies can exert agonist-like effects on the respective target organs; for example, antibodies to TSH receptors can stimulate thyroid secretion, and antibodies to prolactin receptors can stimulate casein synthesis. Autoradiographic studies also indicate that, in addition to conformational changes, hormone binding can also induce alterations in the distribution of receptors, with clustering to form aggregates (so-called 'patches and caps'), which then become internalised (Figure 6.2). The process of internalisation and its consequences appear quite distinct from the immediate events that lead to cell activation; however, the internalisation may still be important in regulating other events, such as new receptor biosynthesis. Internalised receptor sites may be degraded, leading to 'down-regulation' (see below), or may escape degradation and be recycled back for re-insertion into the plasma membrane.

Not only do receptors diffuse freely within the plasma membrane, but they may also pass to intracellular sites for recycling, synthesis and degradation, so that a dynamic equilibrium is set up which may readily be distorted. Thus, the numbers and characteristics of cell surface receptors can be affected by a large number of factors related both to intracellular events and to a variety of extracellular stimuli produced by hormones and other agents. Tachyphylaxis, the decrease in responsiveness of target tissue on continuous or repeated exposure to a hormone, is well known. Functionally, such a response could protect against excessively large rises in hormone concentration. It may be relevant physically in so far as many hormones are secreted episodically, and target cells may be optimally activated by intermittent stimulation. An extreme form of desensitisation is seen following continuous treatment with LHRH agonists, when normal gonadotroph function is inhibited and secretion is suppressed in the face of continued administration of agonist. This form of hormone refractoriness, or 'homologous desensitisation', probably results from changes at the receptor level such as persistent occupancy, inactivation or internalisation of binding sites. Decreases in responsiveness of target cells to a given hormone can also be produced by exposure to other ligands — 'heterologous desensitisation'. Such mechanisms could contribute to developmental changes seen in receptor content and coupling to effector systems.

Down-regulation is not the only way in which receptor numbers may be modulated. In some instances, an increase in receptor numbers may be seen. Thus, under the influence of oestrogens, the number of oxytocin receptors in the uterus increases at the onset of parturition. There are many other instances of regulation by steroids of receptors for peptide hormones, which illustrate the genetic control of receptor content and function. Control may also be localised within the plasma membrane, as in the insulin-mediated binding of insulin-like growth factors, multiplication-stimulating activity (MSA) and basic somatomedin by rat adipocytes. As starvation leads to a fall in insulin levels, this suggests that the effects of the somatomedins may decrease during starvation without changes in the circulating levels.

Important, too, in considering receptor regulation is the concept of 'spare receptors'. In many tissues full occupancy of hormone receptors is not necessary for the full expression of the hormonal response. In such systems, often only 10 to 20 per cent of the total number of receptors present need to be occupied to produce a maximum response of the cell — a reduction in receptor number in such tissues would decrease sensitivity without necessarily changing the maximum possible response. This offers further possibility for control and regulation.

Activation of Adenylate Cyclase

The sequence of molecular events that follow receptor binding leading to elevation of cyclic AMP is fairly well understood, and therefore this system will be described as a model for signal-generating systems. It may well be analogous to the calcium-generating system. The receptor structure responsible for binding the hormone is just one of three functional units which make up the hormone-sensitive adenylate cyclase, the other two being the regulatory protein (N) and the catalytic moeity (C) (Figure 6.3). Whereas the receptor is different for each

Figure 6.3: Binding of Hormone (H) to the Cell Surface Receptor (R) is Followed by Increased Binding of GTP to the Intermediate Nucleotide Regulatory Protein (N) which, in Turn, Causes Activation of the Catalytic Unit (C) Responsible for the Conversion of ATP to Cyclic AMP (cAMP). Binding of cAMP to the regulatory subunit of the inactive protein kinase results in dissociation of the complex and activation of the catalytic subunit. The active protein kinase is rather non-specific with respect to the protein substrate

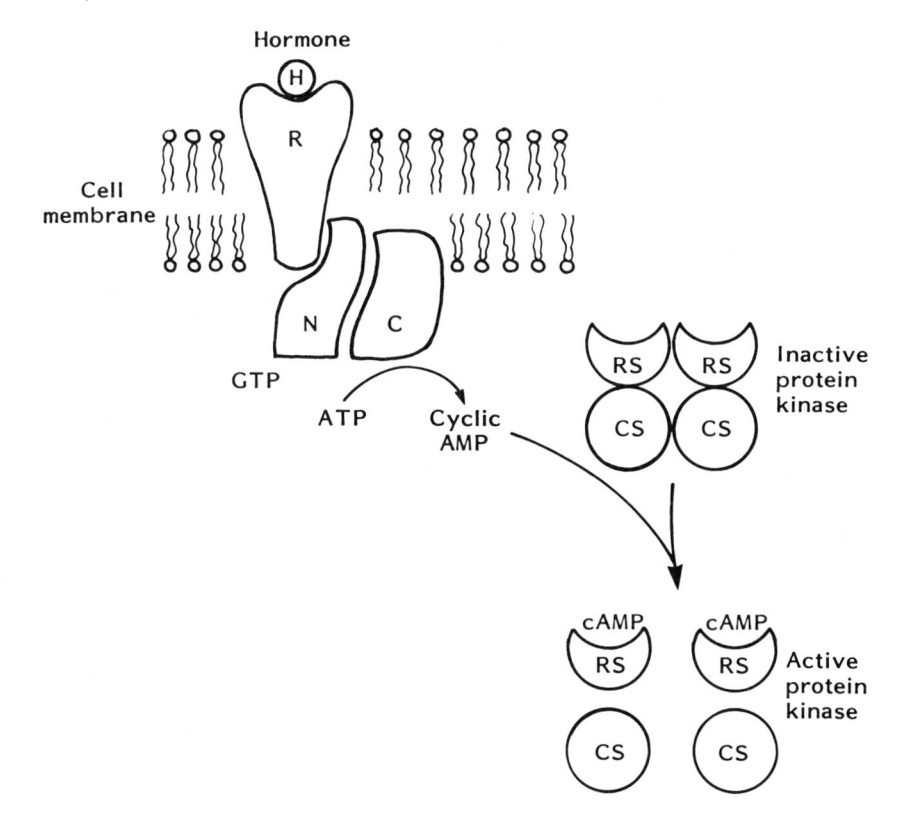

hormone, it appears that activation of the adenylate cyclase moiety is similar for all hormones. Thus it is possible to hybridise receptors with N and C units from other cells and obtain a response. The N binding protein has a molecular weight of 90 000 to 130 000 and comprises two subunits, the larger binding GTP and the smaller interacting with the receptor unit. The C unit also appears to be oligomeric in nature. On binding of the hormone with its receptor, the complex interacts with the smaller subunit of the N protein leading to dissociation of the larger subunit which is then converted to its active form by GTP binding. Subsequently GTP-degrading activity associated with the N protein causes its deactivation by converting bound GTP to GDP and favouring dissociation from the subunit. Upon binding of GTP to N, the C protein is activated and converted from its inactive form to an active one, thereby catalysing the conversion of ATP to cAMP with subsequent stimulation of cell activity. Adenylate cyclases are coupled to hormone receptors in an inhibitory mode as well as a stimulatory mode; study of the inhibition of adenylate cyclase suggests that inhibitory hormones act through a separate GTP binding site which interacts directly with the catalytic unit or uncouples the stimulatory GTP site from the catalytic unit.

Cyclic AMP

The general stimulation of cyclic AMP production by hormones is not as non-specific as it might appear at first sight. As all cells arise by specific differentiation, it is likely that the specificity required by the different cell types is already present in the specific receptor on the cell surface. Secondly, if the intracellular concentration of cyclic AMP is increased by a mechanism not involving hormonal interaction, e.g. administration of exogenous cyclic AMP or inhibition of the enzymes catalysing the destruction of cyclic AMP, then the physiological function of that particular cell is increased. Thus, administration of ACTH *or* of cyclic AMP to an adrenal cell will result in the same effect, i.e. increased steroidogenesis. Thus, the effect of a change in the intracellular concentration depends on the cell type in which the change occurs, i.e. it depends on the process of cellular differentiation.

The discovery of cyclic AMP opened up a whole new chapter in the understanding of mechanisms of hormone action. It has been suggested that a number of criteria should be met before cyclic AMP can be considered to act as the intracellular mediator of the system under study:

(1) that the hormone (or other biological substance, e.g. biogenic amine) should cause an increase in the accumulation of intracellular cyclic AMP in the target tissue;
(2) that the increase in cyclic AMP should precede any change in the physiological response;
(3) that the hormone should activate adenylate cyclase in broken cell (or plasma membrane) preparations;
(4) that inhibitors of phosphodiesterase activity should potentiate the effect of the hormone;
(5) that exogenous cyclic AMP or its analogues should mimic the action of the hormone. (Forskolin, an activator of adenylate cyclase, should also have such effects.)

It has been proposed that all of the biological effects of cyclic AMP are mediated through the activation of protein kinases, which then catalyse the transfer of phosphate from ATP to a protein acceptor. Cyclic AMP-dependent protein kinases are widely distributed in nature, and many proteins other than phosphorylase kinase have been shown to be substrates for these enzymes, including membrane and ribosomal proteins and enzymes. Protein kinases comprise two subunits: a regulatory and a catalytic subunit. The mechanism by which cyclic AMP activates protein kinase is shown in Figure 6.3, and is as follows. While the catalytic subunit is bound to the regulatory subunit, the enzyme is inactive. Cyclic AMP binds to the regulatory subunit, causing the two subunits to dissociate. The free catalytic subunit is then active and able to catalyse the transfer of phosphate to the protein substrate.

To the original criteria may then be added:

(6) that cyclic AMP-dependent protein kinases are present in the cell, and that intracellular activation of these enzymes is observed with hormonal stimulation.

Yet one more way in which cyclic AMP-mediated responses could be brought about is through the involvement of subcellular organelles, the microtubules and microfilaments. Microtubules are linear, unbranched structures of diameter about 25 nm whereas the microfilaments are smaller, fibrous, linear structures about 5 nm in diameter. These structures are thought to be involved in maintaining cell structure and function, in particular those processes in which membrane interactions or movements occur. Cyclic AMP, perhaps via activation of protein kinases, may modulate these processes. Recently it has been shown that following stimulation of cultured thyroid cells with thyrotrophin or cyclic AMP there is a major change in the structure of the microtrabecular lattice, with dissolution of the lattice in the cell periphery and loss of microfilament bundles. Similar effects have been reported in cultured adrenal and ovarian granulosa cells exposed to ACTH or FSH, respectively.

For most hormone systems the intermediate mechanisms between cyclic AMP activation of protein kinase and the response are unknown. One of the most fully investigated systems is the hormonal control of glycogen metabolism.

Glycogenolysis in the liver is stimulated by a number of hormones including adrenaline. An outline of the events that bring about adrenaline stimulation of glycogen breakdown is shown in Figure 6.1. Thus, the protein kinase and its phosphorylated protein form a link in a long chain of events. A simplification of the scheme is to consider the process in three stages: the signal, amplification of the signal, and the effect. The signal is the formation of cAMP, one molecule of hormone stimulating one molecule of cAMP. Phosphorylase *b*-kinase, on the other hand, being an enzyme, can catalyse the transformation of numerous molecules of phosphorylase *b* to the active form, *a*, and so acts to amplify the signal. At the same time as activating phosphorylase kinase, cyclic AMP-dependent protein kinase catalyses the phosphorylation (and in this case inactivation) of glycogen synthetase. Protein kinases in general have important effects on protein synthesis, and are involved in the phosphorylation of nuclear histones and perhaps other nuclear proteins. Consequently RNA synthesis and protein synthesis may be affected.

Cyclic AMP is thus a key intracellular regulator in many hormone-mediated responses. It is an intriguing fact that a metabolic function for cyclic AMP preceded and actually led to its discovery. On the other hand, no clue as to the biological role of a second cyclic nucleotide, cyclic guanosine 5'-monophosphate (GMP), was uncovered until at least seven years after its occurrence was reported. The metabolism of cyclic GMP is similar to cyclic AMP, and cyclic GMP-dependent protein kinases have been found in many tissues. The key observation which provided an insight into the role of cyclic GMP was that acetylcholine-induced depression of cardiac contractility is associated with a relatively rapid accumulation of cyclic GMP. This cholinergic action on cyclic GMP has been observed in a number of tissues, appears to be mediated by muscarinic receptors, and requires the presence of Ca^{++} in the extracellular medium. The cholinergic action on the heart is opposite to that of adrenaline, which elevates myocardial cyclic AMP concentrations. Such evidence has provoked discussion of a possible second-messenger function for this nucleotide. However, the full biological role of cyclic GMP remains to be established. Changes in cyclic GMP levels seem often to be consequences of changes in cytosolic calcium, and cyclic GMP derivatives usually do not mimic the effects of physiological stimuli. Some of the suggested mediators of hypothalamic hormonal control of the pituitary are shown in Table 6.1.

Calcium

In contrast to the cyclic AMP system, where generation of cyclic AMP is nearly always due to direct coupling between hormone and receptor, the change in the calcium signal may not be the initial consequence of hormone receptor activation. From the point of view of transmitting information, the most important factor is the free calcium ion concentration in the cell cytosol. This can be controlled via a cytosolic buffering system and pumps across the plasma, mitochondrial and endoplasmic-reticulum membranes. Hormone binding to receptor causes

Table 6.1: Mediators within the Pituitary Gland of the Action of Hypothalamic Hormones

Hormone	Effect	Mediated by
GnRH	LH ; FSH	Rise in cAMP; increase in cytosol Ca^{++}; ?rise in cGMP
GHRH	GH	Rise in cAMP
TRH	TSH	Rise in cAMP; increase in cytosol Ca^{++}
Somatostatin	GH ; TSH	Fall in cAMP; reduction in cytosol Ca^{++}; ?post-Ca^{++} events
CRF-41	ACTH ; LPH ; etc.	Rise in cAMP
Dopamine	Prolactin	?Fall in cAMP

Note that several processes may be involved for the effects of a given releasing hormone, and that long-term changes in pituitary hormone synthesis may depend on an increase in messenger RNA production. The dopamine receptor was previously thought to act independently of cAMP at the lactotroph, but there is now good evidence that at least part of the process of prolactin inhibition involves a fall in internal cAMP. Increasing work suggests that changes in cytosol Ca^{++} are dependent on alterations in phosphotidyl inositol.

Mechanisms of Peptide Hormone Action 71

Figure 6.4: Postulated Role of Ca^{++} and Phospholipid Turnover in Hormone Action. Cyclic AMP and cyclic GMP may feedback to control the receptor-linked phospholipid degradation (see text).

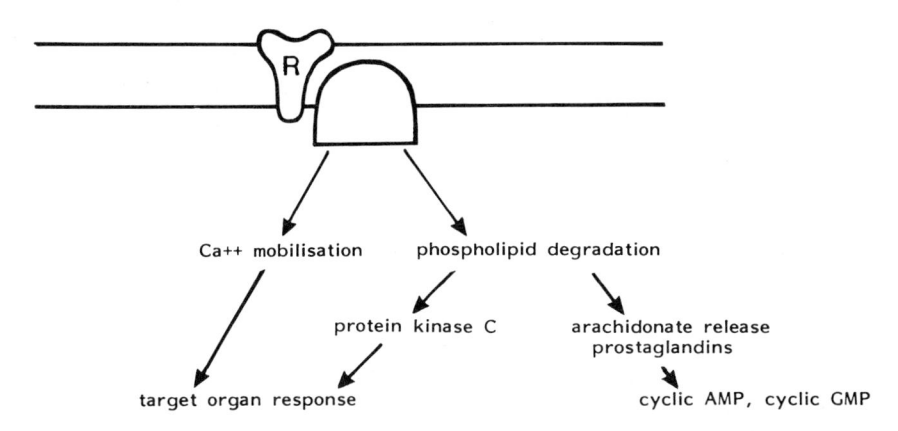

```
─────────────┬──R──┬─────────────
             │     │
             │     │
─────────────┴─────┴─────────────
           /        \
          /          \
  Ca++ mobilisation   phospholipid degradation
    /        \                \
   /      protein kinase C    arachidonate release
  /            /              prostaglandins
 /            /                    ↓
target organ response         cyclic AMP, cyclic GMP
```

mobilisation of calcium by activation of one or more mechanisms. Thus, in many cells, the response appears to be the release of calcium bound to the plasma membrane followed by an increase in the rate of influx through a specific calcium channel. It has also been suggested that important in controlling the rise in cytosolic calcium ions is the breakdown of phosphatidyl inositol, a quantitatively minor anionic phospholipid (Figure 6.4). Release of arachidonic acid and activation of guanylate cyclase are also postulated to play a role. The increase in calcium concentration in the cytosol leads to activation of caldium-dependent enzymes which involve calmodulin as an intermediary (calcium-dependent regulatory protein). This is a calcium receptor present in all mammalian cells. There are at least two mechanisms by which the calmodulin-calcium complex can bring about intracellular changes. In the first, the calmodulin-calcium complex formed as a result of a rise in the calcium ion concentration associates with phosphodiesterase to produce the activated form of the enzyme so that cyclic AMP is controlled indirectly by calcium flux into the cell. In the second system, such as that for phosphorylase kinase, calmodulin represents a subunit of the enzyme. In this instance allosteric modification of the bound subunit by calmodulin leads to a calcium-dependent activation of the enzyme. Thus phosphorylase kinase may be controlled by both cyclic AMP and calcium via calmodulin; this could allow for fine tuning of the secretory process by a variety of local metabolic processes. Whereas the major identified response for cyclic AMP is a change in the state of phosphorylation induced by protein kinase, in the calcium system a number of response elements have been identified, including general and specific protein kinases, calcium transport systems, and microtubule assembly. As well as being indirectly controlled by calcium, cyclic AMP in turn acts at multiple sites to influence calcium messengers. An example of the possible interplay between cyclic AMP and calcium in response to hormone stimulation is given by the model for ACTH. Although it was found that ACTH binding correlated with changes in cyclic AMP concentrations, it was also found that this hormone stimulates steroidogenesis at lower concentrations than those needed to stimulate cyclic AMP concentrations. The mechanisms of action of ACTH have been re-evaluated, and it appears that there are in fact two sets of receptors, one of high affinity and one of low affinity. The range over which ACTH binds to the low-affinity sites is similar to the range over which adenylate cyclase is activated, so it appears that the adenylate cyclase is coupled to these low-affinity receptors whereas calcium ions are linked to the high-affinity receptors.

Hormone Action on Cell Permeability and Protein Synthesis

Although most peptide hormones appear to act via cyclic AMP, several — including insulin, prolactin, growth hormone and growth factors — do not. For these hormones the signal responsible for eliciting cell responses has not been identified. Growth hormone acts by altering membrane permeability and hence the availability of amino acids and energy substrates. It also acts on protein synthesis, appearing to modify the ability of ribosomes to translate messenger RNA into protein synthesis, since the hormone can stimulate protein synthesis in a way not involving an increase in production of messenger RNA. In the stimulation of protein synthesis, hormone-induced peptide messengers may be involved, derived from the receptor or by activation of an intrinsic membrane protein. Thus, in the mammary gland, prolactin stimulates the formation of a plasma membrane factor that enhances casein messenger RNA formation in the nucleus. Another recent finding of importance with respect to the action of hormones such as insulin and the epidermal growth factor is phosphorylation of the receptor molecule. For example, ligand-stimulated phosphorylation of the epidermal growth factor receptor occurs during hormone binding, and is mainly confined to tyrosine residues rather than serine or threonine residues.

Like growth hormone, insulin has an effect on cell permeability. Thus enhanced transfer of glucose and amino acids into the cell is the primary effect of insulin. Much research has been carried out into the kinetics and characteristics of the insulin receptors, but the action of insulin in modifying membrane transport properties is not fully understood; however, insulin may mask or unmask some component of the membrane which is involved in such transport, and thus increase its efficiency. This transport is thought to involve a carrier molecule in the membrane. Transport into the cell of substances such as glucose is best explained in terms of a mobile carrier. The criteria for carrier-mediated transfer are as follows:

(1) The transfer should occur more rapidly than simple diffusion.
(2) The transfer process should exhibit saturation kinetics, i.e. the system should be saturated at a given concentration of the substance transported.
(3) Competition with similar molecules should be demonstrated.
(4) It should also be possible to demonstrate inhibition with certain agents, e.g. those acting with sulphydryl groups.

(5) It should be possible to demonstrate counter-flow, i.e. the movement of a previously accumulated substrate out of the cell when a different substrate is added to the medium.

An insulin-sensitive sugar transport process exists in many cells, including those of skeletal and cardiac muscle and adipose tissue. Similar insulin-sensitive carrier mechanisms also exist for certain amino acids. Associated with these transport phenomena are ion fluxes, for example, of potassium and magnesium.

Receptors and Disease

At present there are relatively few diseases attributable to a deficiency in the number or function of hormone receptors. The spectrum of such diseases could cover under- or overproduction of receptors, altered receptor affinity, antireceptor antibodies, or abnormal receptor-effector coupling.

The occurrence of hormone-secreting pituitary adenomas may be due to altered receptor concentration. Thus, one of the proposed causes of prolactin-secreting pituitary adenomas is a loss of or severe reduction in the dopamine-receptor population in the mammotroph. On the other hand, receptor overproduction may be involved as a contributory factor in pituitary adenomas responsible for Cushing's disease and acromegaly. However, the responsiveness of prolactinomas both *in vivo* and *in vitro* (see Figure 7.1) to dopamine agonist therapy suggests that, at least qualitatively, the lactotroph dopamine receptors are intact. More detailed studies have suggested that a partial resistance of dopamine receptors may exist in microprolactinomas, but these studies require confirmation. Similarly, although some patients with Cushing's disease respond with excessive ACTH responses to CRF-41, many do not, which argues against a primary abnormality in the CRF receptor. Recent data indicate that 'normal' GH responses to GHRH are also not infrequently seen in acromegaly. The changes in receptor concentration are well documented for several forms of insulin resistance and in type LL hypercholesterolaemia with decreased low-density lipoprotein receptors. There is a receptor-related defect in a variant of pseudohypoparathyroidism in which the defect lies not in the PTH receptor itself, but apparently in the subunit responsible for coupling receptor occupancy to activation of adenylate cyclase.

The best-characterised disorders affecting receptors are those that result from the presence of autoantibodies which can react with the receptors. They act as competitive antagonists or exert destructive effects, as in myasthenia gravis, or as agonists producing persistent stimulation, as seen in Graves' disease. In this latter condition thyroid stimulating immunoglobulins are present. It is of interest that, in patients with adrenergic hyper-responsiveness, antibodies against adrenergic receptors were discovered as a result of a deliberate search for such immunoglobulins.

A great deal is known about the TSH receptor and its diseases. Most significant are the secondary diseases resulting from antibodies, although two congenital forms have been described, an isolated thyroid variety and that associated with pseudohypoparathyroidism as described earlier. Graves' and Hashimoto's diseases are both autoimmune diseases, the nature of the disease depending on the predominating immune product. When thyroid stimulating antibodies predominate, Graves' disease is seen. Where destructive antibodies are predominantly secreted, thyroid cells become destroyed, with the thyroid features of Hashimoto's disease. Many assays for thyroid stimulating antibodies have been developed, the most practical techniques employing generation of cyclic AMP by TSH or thyroid stimulating antibodies as the end-point of bioassays *in vitro*. It should be noted that generation of cyclic AMP by the cell in the presence of TSH-receptor antibodies is still not equivalent to the demonstration of thyroid hormone release, which is best shown by changes in thyroid activity in the mouse *in vivo* assay. However, the latter technique is tedious and expensive, and more rapid techniques for clinical use are still being investigated. Receptor binding assays are still further dissociated from the biological end-point of thyroid stimulation. Indeed, these assays reveal that 10-15 per cent of patients with autoimmune thyroiditis have detectable thyroid binding inhibitory activity. The ability to secrete thyroid antibodies appears to be inherited in a significant proportion of the population, but they are usually only important if present in high titre. Recently it has been suggested that in many cases of Hashimoto's thyroiditis the goitre is due to growth-stimulating antibodies rather than to a compensatory excess TSH drive.

As far as application of knowledge of the receptor response is concerned, an important observation is the ability of GnRH agonists to desensitise the pituitary gland and to inhibit gonadotrophin secretion. To induce fertility, LHRH has to be given in a pulsatile fashion. The receptor-mediated desensitisation of the pituitary by LHRH agonists has been used clinically in situations in which suppression of the gonadotrophins is of value, as in the treatment of idiopathic precocious puberty, metastatic breast cancer, prostatic cancer and endometriosis.

As yet, little is known of the way in which defects in the intracellular mechanisms of hormone action contribute to altered function. It is possible, however, to gain some information as to the site at which a block may occur. Thus lithium, which produces nephrogenic diabetes insipidus, has been postulated to influence cyclic AMP concentrations in the vasopressin-sensitive renal tubule cells and possibly to act at a point beyond the formation of cyclic AMP. Understanding of intracellular mechanisms in hormone responses may thus provide a fruitful area for future investigation of disease.

Further Reading

Adams, D.D. (1980) 'Thyroid-stimulating Autoantibodies', *Vitamins and Hormones, 38*, 120-203

Canonico, P.L. and MacLeod, R.M. (1983) 'The Role of Phospholipids in Hormonal Secretory Mechanisms', in E.E. Muller and R.M. MacLeod (eds), *Neuroendocrine Perspectives*, vol. 2, pp. 123-72, Elsevier, Amsterdam

Catt, K.J. and Dufau, M.L. (1983) 'Clinical Significance of Peptide Hormone Receptors', *Clinics in Endocrinology and Metabolism, 12*, xi-xlv

Greengard, P. (1978) *Cyclic Nucleotides. Phosphorylated Proteins and Neuronal Function*, Raven Press, New York

King, A.C. and Cuatrecasas, P. (1981) 'Peptide Hormone-induced Receptor Mobility Aggregation and Internalization', *New England Journal of Medicine, 305*, 77–88

Levitzki, A. (1982) 'Activation and Inhibition of Adenylate Cyclase by Hormones: Mechanistic Aspects', in J.W. Lamble (ed.), *More about Receptors*, pp. 14–28, Elsevier Biomedical Press, Amsterdam

Nishizuki, Y., Takai, Y., Kishimoto, A., Kikkawa, U. and Kaibuchi, K. (1984) 'Phospholipid Turnover in Hormone Action', *Recent Progress in Hormone Research, 40*, 301–45

Posner, B.I., Bergeron, J.M., Josefsberg, Z., Khan, N., Khan, R.J., Patel, B.A., Sikstrom, R.A. and Verma, A.K. (1981) 'Polypeptide Hormones, Intracellular Receptors and Internalisation', *Recent Progress in Hormone Research, 37*, 539–82

Rasmussen, H. and Waisman, D. (1981) 'The Messenger Function of Calcium in Endocrine Systems', *Biochemical Actions of Hormones, VIII*, 1–115

7 PROLACTIN

Introduction

An effect of the anterior pituitary on lactation was first reported in 1928. Shortly afterwards it was found that extracts of bovine pituitaries stimulated mammary gland development in the rat. Prolactin was first purified in 1955 and was shown to have effects on the secretion of the pigeon crop, to have luteotrophic effects in rodents, and to influence osmoregulation in amphibians. Human prolactin is, like growth hormone, a single-chain polypeptide, and the entire linear sequence of 198 amino acids of human prolactin has been determined. It is very similar in structure to human placental lactogen and growth hormone. Indeed, growth hormone and prolactin are so similar that at one time it was believed that the human pituitary contained no prolactin. To this day the complete role of prolactin in human physiology is still rather an enigma. Native human prolactin, like other polypeptide hormones (such as insulin, growth hormone and parathyroid hormone), is not one single molecular species, but is heterogeneous. Polymers of prolactin molecules appear to be precursor or storage forms, and are normally only secreted in small amounts. However, in states of high secretion rates, such as in pregnancy or idiopathic galactorrhoea, more of these 'big' molecules may appear in the circulation. Although primarily produced in the lactotroph, extrapituitary production from other brain areas, placental tissues and neoplastic tissues has been reported.

Assay of Prolactin

Until very recently, bioassays of prolactin have relied either on the proliferative action of the hormone on the mucosal epithelium of pigeons, or on the stimulation of mammary growth or lactation in mammals. Normally, *in vitro* assays employing mouse mammary gland explants are used, the effect of prolactin being determined either histologically or biochemically: the parameters measured are the appearance of milk, enzyme induction or casein synthesis. A highly sensitive bioassay has recently been described which exploits the observation that the growth of cell cultures derived from Nb 2 lymphomas in the rat is stimulated by very small quantities of prolactin. Growth hormone has a similar effect, but cross-reaction can be prevented by incubating the assay samples with growth hormone antiserum. Growth hormone can, of course, also be estimated in this system.

This bioassay is more sensitive than the radioimmunoassays that have been developed for the measurement of prolactin from various species. Although radioimmunoassays for human prolactin are now in widespread use, they are not totally satisfactory since purified human prolactin for use as standard, as material for iodination or immunogen, is difficult to prepare. However, RIAs are now the routine method for measuring prolactin, with bioassays available in some centres to investigate apparent discrepancies between biochemical and biological activity.

During the last few years radioreceptor assays for prolactin have also been developed. These rely on the binding of prolactin to specific receptors on mammary epithelial cells.

Control of Prolactin

The normal range of circulating prolactin concentration is around 100–360 mU/litre (5–18 ng/ml), although higher concentrations are observed in certain situations, for example pregnancy (see later). The biological half-life of prolactin is similar to that of growth hormone, being around 30 min. Although in many species prolactin is a major constituent of the anterior pituitary, this is not the case in man, where there is around 100 μg of prolactin per pituitary, which is less than in other species.

Suckling is the most potent physiological stimulus for prolactin secretion. Stimulation of the breast (or, more particularly, the nipple) at other times, e.g. during sexual activity, also results in increased prolactin release. Sensory receptors in the breast initiate neural impulses which reach the hypothalamus. Pregnancy is not a prerequisite for this reflex. Over the course of pregnancy, prolactin concentrations increase to 10 to 20 times the non-pregnant values. This rise is related to the increase in circulating oestrogens. Intravenous and intra-amniotic administration of a precursor of oestradiol in pregnancy results in elevated prolactin concentrations. Oestradiol may influence the secretion of prolactin either by a direct action on the pituitary, where a major action appears to be stimulation of protein synthesis, or by a more complex action at the level of the hypothalamus. If the mother does not suckle the baby post-partum, the prolactin concentrations rapidly decrease, and normalise in 2 to 6 weeks. With breast-feeding, however, the serum prolactin remains elevated; there is a very gradual decline over many months, with superimposed bursts associated with suckling.

During the latter half of gestation, serum prolactin concentrations in the fetus are markedly elevated. They fall at birth to a slightly elevated level, which is maintained for about six weeks, and thereafter fall to prepubertal levels. In girls there is a small rise prior to menarche and a further rise post-menarche. There are variations in serum prolactin according to the phase of the menstrual cycle, but the absolute magnitude of these changes is very small.

Basal prolactin levels show fluctuations suggesting an episodic secretory pattern. During sleep the amplitude of these fluctuations increases. This night-time elevation in circulating prolactin is dependent on sleep, and not on an innate rhythm; excursions are maximal during 'slow-wave' or non-dreaming sleep. Both physical and psychic (e.g. anxiety) stress are said to result in an increase in circulating prolactin although the evidence for such an effect is not wholly conclusive.

Mediators of Prolactin Release

Regulation of prolaction secretion by the hypothalamus is predominantly inhibitory. This became apparent many years ago through experiments in which stalk secretion, ectopic pituitary grafts, hypothalamic lesions and *in vitro* incubation of adrenohypophysial tissue resulted in *increased* prolactin secretion. It was postulated that, *in vivo*, a prolactin inhibiting factor (PIF) was released from the median eminence into the portal vessels, resulting in an inhibition of prolactin release from the lactotroph cells.

There is still some uncertainty as to the true nature of PIF (or PIFs). In man, a number of drugs that influence dopaminergic mechanisms also affect prolactin secretion. For example, L-dopa, which increases dopamine production in the hypothalamus, and bromocriptine, an ergot derivative acting as a dopamine receptor agonist, inhibit prolactin secretion. Dopamine and bromocriptine act directly on the prolactin-secreting cells in a dose-dependent manner (Figure 7.1). Furthermore, dopamine antagonists (neuroleptics) cause an increase in prolactin secretion *in vivo* and *in vitro*. Dopamine receptors have been found on pituitary cells,

Figure 7.1: Control of Prolactin Release Shown by a Human Prolactinoma *in vitro*. The tumour cells were dispersed with trypsin and then perfused with dopamine and then bromocriptine. Persistent inhibition of prolactin is shown in the presence of bromocriptine. (A. Grossman, G. Delitala and G.M. Besser, unpublished observations.)

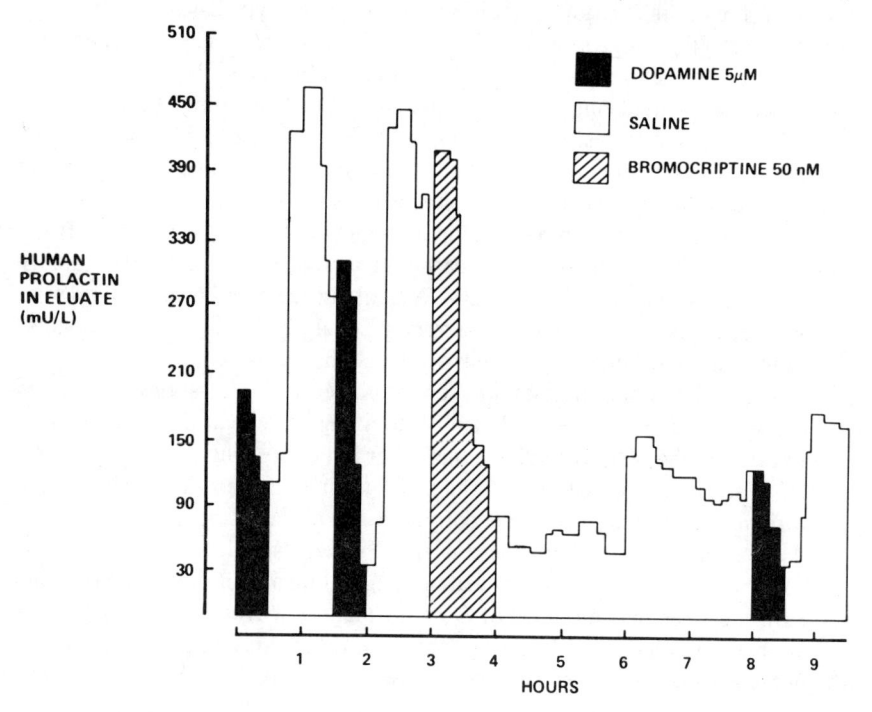

and more recently dopamine has been detected in portal blood in a concentration sufficient to inhibit prolactin release significantly. It appears that this catecholamine reaches the pituitary from tubero-infundibular neurones which terminate in the median eminence adjacent to the portal vessels.

Although it is clear that dopamine is a major PIF, there is still uncertainty as to whether another non-dopaminergic PIF exists. Dopamine does account for most, but not all, of the PIF activity present in the mediobasal hypothalamus. Certain catecholamine-free extracts of medial basal hypothalamus retain some residual PIF activity. In addition, the concentrations of dopamine measured in the hypophysial stalk plasma will not completely suppress spontaneous prolactin release. There have been suggestions that γ-aminobutyric acid (GABA) might be a PIF, but it is about two orders of magnitude less potent than dopamine. Whether the concentration of portal blood GABA is physiologically significant remains highly controversial (Figure 7.2).

Figure 7.2: Hypothalamic Mechanisms Controlling Prolactin Release. See text for details

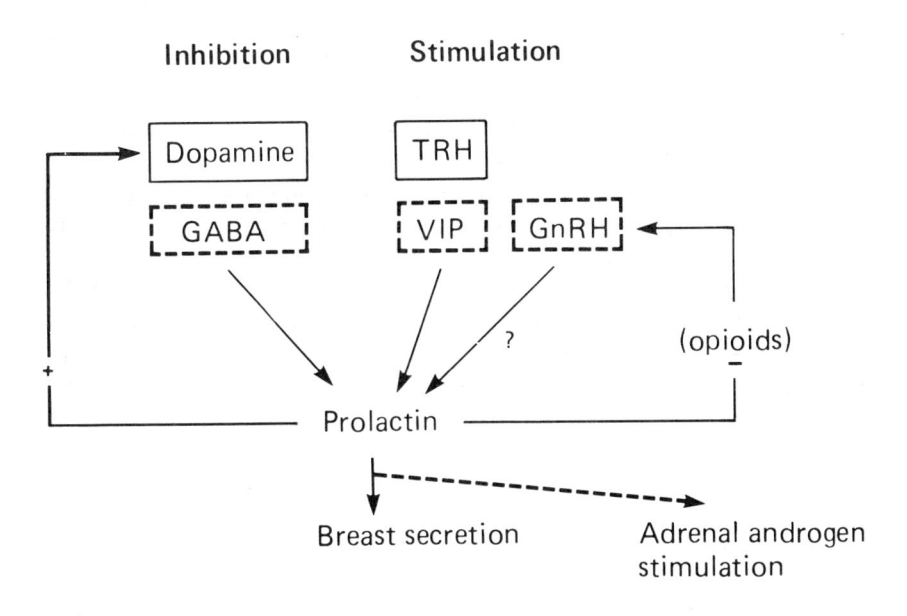

Very recently, the genomic sequence of the precursor to LHRH has been determined, and includes a peptide which has potent prolactin-inhibitory activity. The physiological role for this putative hypothalamic hormone remains to be established.

In addition to PIF, the hypothalamus may secrete prolactin releasing factor(s). In some animals (including man) thyrotrophin releasing hormone (TRH) causes the release of prolactin. However, TRH may not be the only prolactin-releasing factor under physiological conditions since the question of whether the suckling stimulus increases TSH secretion is a matter of debate. The effect of suckling on prolactin secretion may, at least in part, be mediated by a decrease in the PIF concentration reaching the pituitary, but there is evidence that this does not account for the total release of prolactin seen.

Other putative modulators of prolactin secretion are serotonin, the endogenous opiate agonists, and several of the brain-gut peptides, especially VIP (vasoactive intestinal peptide) . Inhibition of serotonin synthesis blocks suckling-induced prolactin response, and endorphins (including methionine-enkephalin) cause increased prolactin release. In the rat, the specific receptor antagonist naloxone reduces basal, suckling-induced and stress-related release of prolactin, but there is little evidence that endogenous opioids are important physiological regulators of prolactin release in man.

Prolactin also exerts an inhibitory control over its own secretion; this is thought to be mediated by dopamine via the tubero-infundibular neurones. Ectopic pituitary transplantation leads to both increased prolactin release and increased dopamine release, and the administration of a prolactin-stimulating drug increases hypothalamic dopamine synthesis; furthermore, the suckling reflex which results in increased prolactin secretion also leads to a decrease in the dopamine content of the hypothalamus.

Of the brain-gut peptides, VIP is a possible candidate as a physiological prolactin-releasing factor. Receptors for VIP are found on pituitary membranes, and VIP uptake in the pituitary appears to be exclusively localised to lactotrophs. The peptide is present in the hypothalamus and hypophysial portal system, but relatively large concentrations are required to stimulate release. Infusion of VIP in man has been shown to stimulate prolactin release.

The list of drugs that enhance prolactin secretion is a growing one. It includes major tranquillisers, e.g. phenothiazines and thioxanthines, antihypertensives such as α-methyldopa and reserpine, antiemetics such as metoclopramide, the histamine-2 receptor antagonist cimetidine (only at high intravenous doses), oestrogen (as in oral contraceptives) and opiates. Further details are given in Table 7.1.

Actions of Prolactin

The primary action of prolactin is to stimulate lactation. A number of hormones, including oestrogen, progesterone, GH, adrenal steroids, insulin, thyroid hormones and prolactin, are involved in mammary-gland develpoment. During pregnancy, prolactin levels begin to rise in the first trimester and increase progressively until term. There is a synergism between corticosteroids and prolactin on lactogenesis, so that the parallel increases in these hormones around parturition appear to be of considerable importance. During pregnancy the combined effects of prolactin, human placental lactogen, oestrogens and progesterone develop the secretory apparatus of the breast but do not allow lactation. It seems

Table 7.1: Causes of Hyperprolactinaemia

Prolactinomas: Small and large

Lesions of hypothalamus and pituitary stalk:
    functionless tumours
    acromegaly
    Cushing's syndrome
    hypothalamic tumours and granulomas, e.g. craniopharyngiomas, neurosarcoidosis, histiocytosis X, germinomas
    empty sella syndrome
    cranial radiotherapy
    trauma

Primary hypothyroidism

Renal failure

Drugs:
    major tranquillisers, e.g. butyrophenones (haloperidol); phenothiazines (chlorpromazine)
    antiemetics, e.g. metoclopramide, domperidone
    antihypertensives, e.g. reserpine, methyldopa
    TRH
    opiates

Chest-wall lesions:
    trauma
    herpes zoster

Idiopathic/functional
    hypovolaemia and some forms of stress, including hypoglycaemia, stimulate prolactin release transiently

likely that oestrogen is inhibitory to milk secretion and that the fall in this steroid near parturition is the trigger for lactation, that is, the lactogenic action of prolactin is then unopposed. Furthermore, progesterone appears to inhibit prolactin secretion, and so the fall in progesterone levels may also be responsible for the pre-partum increase in circulating prolactin concentrations. During lactation basal prolactin is not particularly high, but rises dramatically when the young suckle. Lactation may continue for long periods as long as nursing occurs. Prolactin and adrenal steroids are both essential for the initiation and maintenance of lactation. Hypophysectomy in experimental animals results in an immediate cessation of milk secretion, whereas adrenalectomy leads to a more progressive reduction in secretion.

    Prolactin interacts with receptors in the mammary gland but, unlike many other peptide hormones, its action does not appear to be mediated via changes in cyclic nucleotide metabolism. Whatever the second messenger for prolactin, it seems that the cytoskeleton is important, as disruption of the microtubule system reduces the response to prolactin. Subsequent to binding of prolactin there is an increase in the synthesis of messenger, ribosomal and transfer RNA and in the synthesis of milk proteins (e.g. casein and lactalbumin) and of enzymes (e.g. galactosyl transferase). The effects on the mammary glands are not confined to milk protein synthesis. Prolactin stimulates synthesis of lactose and medium-chain fatty acids, and has a marked effect on ion transport.

It has long been known that ovulation is delayed in nursing mothers, indicating an inhibitory effect of prolactin on the hypothalamo-pituitary-gonadal axis. High serum prolactin levels are associated with decreased LH and FSH concentrations and the normal episodic secretion of LH is inhibited although the response to LHRH is unimpaired. This suggests an inhibition of the pulsatile release of hypothalamic GnRH, which has been demonstrated directly in the rat. It appears that endogenous opioids, probably β-endorphin, are involved in this process. High prolactin also has an inhibitory effect on the ovaries, in that they appear to be less responsive to FSH under these conditions.

A wide variety of other actions have been ascribed to prolactin in different species. An osmoregulatory function has been suggested in certain fish and amphibians, but there is controversy as to whether this is an important function in mammals. Furthermore, it is still uncertain as to whether prolactin functions as a regulator of fetal or neonatal growth in mammals. In addition, a direct effect of prolactin on the CNS centres controlling sexual drives (libido) is considered likely.

Disorders of Prolactin Secretion

Deficiency of prolactin secretion is rarely seen clinically, hyperprolactinaemia occurring far more frequently. Hypoprolactinaemia may occur in association with pituitary apoplexy or infarction. Probably the only occasion on which prolactin deficiency is a cause for concern is in Sheehan's syndrome, which is seen after severe post-partum haemorrhage and in which lactation does not occur. Since serum prolactin may be very low ($<$ 60 mU/litre), even in normal subjects, prolactin deficiency can only be diagnosed when an undetectable serum prolactin fails to rise after TRH.

It should be realised that serum prolactin is released in a pulsatile fashion from the anterior pituitary gland, and is a 'stress' hormone. Although the latter is rather ill-defined, there is certainly evidence that surgical stress can lead to a considerable elevation of serum prolactin, and syncopal attacks during venepuncture may also produce hyperprolactinaemia. Acute exercise may also lead to a modest elevation in serum prolactin, and food-related rises have been reported. Although the influence of mental stress remains uncertain, it seems reasonable to measure serum prolactin in recumbent and relaxed patients, and to ensure that the patient has not recently undertaken heavy exertion or eaten a large meal. Thus, a single apparently elevated serum prolactin should not be used to define hyperprolactinaemia. Although for these and more technical reasons regarding the prolactin assay, some authorities only regard serum prolactin as truly elevated when above 1000 mU/litre, most neuroendocrinologists regard a persisting serum prolactin above 400 mU/litre as pathological. The most common causes include medication, hypothyroidism, renal failure and hypothalamo-pituitary disease (Table 7.1).

Drugs

Table 7.1 lists the drugs most usually associated with hyperprolactinaemia. The most important group are the major tranquillisers. It has been suggested that the antipsychotic activity of these drugs resides in their dopamine-receptor blockade; if this is so, treatment of concurrent hyperprolactinaemia with bromocriptine might be expected to also antagonise the therapeutic efficacy of these agents. Although this has not been formally tested, it would seem reasonable to try to avoid treating tranquilliser-induced hyperprolactinaemia unless this appears essential. In the latter situation, the minimal dose of bromocriptine necessary to normalise serum prolactin should be used. Long-term high-dose treatment with these drugs may lead to a fall in serum prolactin, and it has been suggested that these agents may also interfere with the lactotroph's secretory apparatus through an interaction with calmodulin. Certain antiemetic drugs such as metoclopramide and domperidone are also dopamine antagonists, and it is important to realise that treatment of bromocriptine-related nausea with these agents is irrational as the therapeutic effect of bromocriptine is thereby lost. Reserpine and methyldopa may induce hyperprolactinaemia by depleting central dopamine stores, but where this is problematic the addition of bromocriptine will not only normalise serum prolactin but may also improve the control of hypertension.

Neither cimetidine nor ranitidine increase serum prolactin in normal therapeutic doses, although large parenteral doses of cimetidine may cause transient hyperprolactinaemia. Opiate alkaloids such as morphine and pentazocine are potent prolactin secretagogues. Oestrogen therapy, as in the combination oral contraceptive, may induce hyperprolactinaemia in certain predisposed individuals; however, analysis of large series of women before and after treatment with the 'pill' suggests that this complication of therapy must be relatively rare. Nevertheless, no woman with untreated hyperprolactinaemia should be treated with the oral contraceptive without thorough investigation, as there is a risk that oestrogen may stimulate the growth of a prolactin-secreting tumour.

Hypothyroidism

Approximately 10 to 20 per cent of patients with primary hypothyroidism may demonstrate hyperprolactinaemia, and may in fact present with menstrual irregularity or even amenorrhoea and galactorrhoea. It has been thought that this is secondary to an elevation in hypothalamic TRH stimulating both TSH and prolactin release. However, it is then difficult to explain why hyperprolactinaemia is not seen in all such patients. Another possible explanation is that the feedback increase in TSH leads to an enlargement of the pituitary and embarrassment of the portal microcirculation in those 10 per cent of patients known (from postmortem histology surveys) to harbour microscopic microadenomas. This would then allow these small prolactinomas to enlarge. Whatever the case, it is certainly true that in many patients with primary hypothyroidism, an elevated serum prolactin may ultimately normalise on treatment with thyroid replacement therapy alone (although this may take many months).

Renal Failure

Hyperprolactinaemia is not infrequently seen in patients with chronic renal failure. Although this is at least partly due to a decrease in clearance of serum prolactin, there is well-substantiated evidence that prolactin production is increased due to a change in lactotroph dopamine-receptor function. The treatment of such patients with bromocriptine will usually normalise serum prolactin, with a cure of the clinical features due to hyperprolactinaemia (see below). Recent studies have also suggested that dietary zinc supplementation may be effective.

Miscellaneous

Elevated serum prolactin has been reported to occur in a high percentage of patients with Hodgkin's disease, but the reason for this association is unknown. Although changes occur in mean serum prolactin in the very old, they do not usually lie outside the normal range and should not cause diagnostic confusion.

There is a largely uncharted area of the effects of psychotropic drugs other than the major tranquillisers on serum prolactin. Monoamine oxidase inhibitors may elevate serum prolactin, but usually not to any significant degree; benzodiazepines have been reported to suppress serum prolactin, possibly through an activation of GABA receptors; tricyclic antidepressants probably do not alter circulating prolactin, although the new agent nomifensine (a dopamine reuptake inhibitor) lowers serum prolactin. In an individual in whom hyperprolactinaemia is suspected as being drug related, there is often little choice but to remeasure prolactin when the patient is off therapy, in order to establish the cause of the hyperprolactinaemia.

Hypothalamo-pituitary Disease

Perhaps the most common aetiology for hyperprolactinaemia is a pituitary prolactin-secreting microadenoma. Because prolactin secretion is tonically inhibited by the hypothalamus, any local abnormality in the region of the normal pituitary lactotrophs may lead to hyperprolactinaemia, even when pituitary tumours do not themselves actually secrete prolactin. Many diagnostic tests have been devised to differentiate 'functional hyperprolactinaemia' from a true microadenoma, but they are unreliable and of little value in the individual patient. Such tests have included stimulation with TRH or a dopamine antagonist such as metoclopramide, or inhibition by an indirectly acting dopamine agonist such as nomifensine. Although patients whose serum prolactin is unresponsive to such tests may usually be shown to harbour a pituitary microadenoma, a positive response to these tests is said *ipso facto* to exclude a tumour, such that no tissue for histology is obtained. With the use of the modern generation of computerised tomography (CT) scanners, small tumours are being directly revealed in many such cases of 'functional' hyperprolactinaemia. Furthermore, it would be surprising if the occasional misdiagnosis did not allow some cases of functional hyperprolactinaemia to come to surgery, but in fact lactotroph hyperplasia is an exceedingly rare finding. Pituitary tumours are discussed in greater detail in Chapter 13.

Some pituitary tumours which undoubtedly do not secrete prolactin cause mild hyperprolactinaemia by tumour compression of the portal vasculature to neighbouring lactotrophs. Similarly, hypothalamic mass lesions, which are uncommon causes of hyperprolactinaemia, may disrupt the normal portal delivery of dopamine to the pituitary. In such cases serum prolactin may only be mildly elevated (< 1000 mU/litre), but levels considerably above this can occasionally be seen with hypothalamic disease. Arachnoid fibrosis following meningo-encephalitis may also cause hyperprolactinaemia by interference with the portal venous system, and non-penetrating injuries to the head may shear these fragile vessels.

Polycystic Ovary Syndrome (PCOS)

Many women with hyperprolactinaemia may eventually be diagnosed as having the polycystic ovary syndrome. The PCOS consists of the classic triad of hirsuties, obesity, and oligomenorrhoea/infertility, previously referred to as the Stein-Leventhal syndrome. However, it should be noted that not all components are necessary for diagnosis, and indeed the presence of polycystic ovaries may be the *consequence* rather than the cause of the hyperandrogenisation. Levels of circulating androgens (e.g. testosterone, androstenedione, and particularly dehydroepiandrosterone sulphate) are elevated, and that of the androgen binding protein sex hormone binding globulin (SHBG) is characteristically low. The source of these excess androgens remains disputed, but both adrenal and ovarian origins have been variously considered predominant. Mild hyperprolactinaemia is seen in approximately 30 per cent of cases. The aetiology of the syndrome is unknown, but the earlier suggestion of a *forme fruste* of congenital adrenal hyperplasia is now generally thought improbable. There is characteristically a high ratio of serum LH/FSH in this condition, and LH pulses of high frequency and amplitude are seen. It is possible that the high LH increases aromatisation of androstenedione to oestrone (a process also accelerated by excess adipose tissue), which in turn stimulates hyperprolactinaemia. Alternatively, prolactin may itself increase the secretion of adrenal androgens, thus setting in train a vicious cycle of positive feedback. Whatever the case, women with PCOS and hyperprolactinaemia may benefit from suppression of their serum prolactin, and a therapeutic trial with bromocriptine is often useful.

Manifestations of Hyperprolactinaemia

In women, significant hyperprolactinaemia is usually associated with secondary amenorrhoea. Galactorrhoea is said to be present in 30 per cent of such cases, although careful examination will often reveal a breast discharge (not always obviously milk-like) in 70 to 80 per cent of patients. Less marked degrees of hyperprolactinaemia cause menstrual irregularity, usually oligomenorrhoea, or occasionally regular menses with an inadequate luteal phase. It is therefore important to measure the serum prolactin in any patient being investigated for infertility. Hyperprolactinaemia is also thought to cause a disturbance of mood and libido, and it is teleologically reasonable for a lactating woman in the puerperium to be rather introverted and lacking in sexual desire. However, the evidence for such changes, as well as that for the association between hyperprolactinaemia and obesity, remains predominantly anecdotal. The suppression of hypothalamic LHRH, and the direct inhibition of ovarian activity, may lead to a profound lowering of serum oestradiol. Hot flushes are not seen, but other symptoms associated with oestrogen deficiency, such as superficial dyspareunia, are seen relatively frequently. Hyperprolactinaemia may (rarely) cause primary amenorrhoea, with evidence of arrested or delayed puberty. Of course, hyperprolactinaemia secondary to a pituitary adenoma may also present with headache or visual defects due to local compressive effects.

In male patients, hyperprolactinaemia causes erectile failure (impotence), but it is *not* associated with either gynaecomastia or oligospermia. In fact, a reduction in seminal fluid volume will often produce an apparent increase in spermatozoa concentration. The impotence may be secondary to pituitary hypogonadotrophism contingent upon actual tumour invasion, or a direct suppression of Leydig cell testosterone production. However, most usually serum testosterone is at the lower end but still within the normal range, and it has been suggested that prolactin inhibits the conversion of testosterone to dihydrotestosterone by the enzyme 5α-reductase. Men presenting with hyperprolactinaemia, in contrast to women, usually have large pituitary tumours; hyperprolactinaemia is an uncommon cause of impotence in surveys of men presenting to sexual dysfunction clinics.

In summary, in female patients presenting with menstrual irregularity or infertility, or in male patients presenting with sexual dysfunction, the diagnosis of hyperprolactinaemia should always be considered.

Treatment of Hyperprolactinaemia

Providing the underlying cause cannot itself be eradicated (such as hypothyroidism), the primary medical treatment in all cases of hyperprolactinaemia is dopamine-agonist therapy. The most widely used dopamine agonist is the ergot alkaloid bromocriptine (2-bromo-α-ergocryptine), but other longer-acting, and hopefully cheaper, preparations (such as pergolide) are being developed (Figure 7.3). Bromocriptine is a highly potent dopamine agonist and its clinical efficacy relates to this pharmacological action. It is extremely effective in suppressing circulating prolactin, regardless of cause, and failures of treatment usually relate to inadequacies in the mode of prescription. The drug has been shown to directly inhibit secretion by the pituitary lactotroph through stimulation of dopamine receptors, and its action is blocked by dopamine antagonists. High circulating levels of bromocriptine are attained by oral medication, and the drug is, for the most part, metabolised rather than excreted intact.

Bromocriptine may cause nausea and postural hypotension when treatment is started, principally through activation of central receptors. These side-effects can always be minimised, and usually totally eliminated, by careful adherence to a scheme for initiation of therapy and by insisting that the drug be taken during

Figure 7.3: Structure of the Dopamine Agonists Bromocriptine and Pergolide

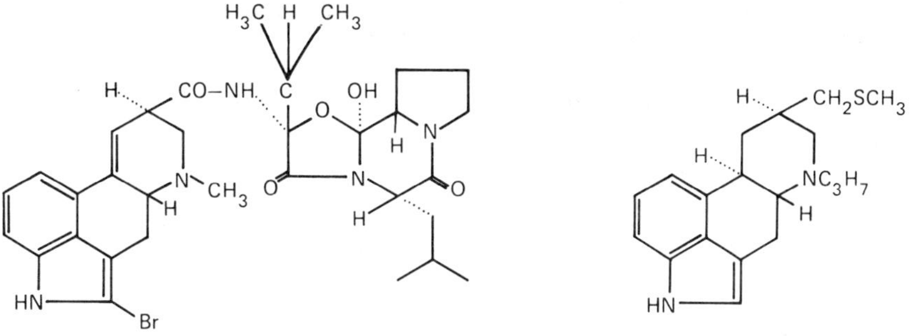

BROMOCRIPTINE   PERGOLIDE

a meal. The first dose is 1.25 mg (half a tablet) should be given at night in the middle of a small snack, such as a sandwich and a glass of milk, as the patient goes to bed. After three or four days this dose is increased to one tablet (2.5 mg) on retiring, and a few days later this dose is moved forward to the middle of the evening meal. The medication is increased at approximately three-day intervals to 2.5 mg twice or three times daily, ensuring that the tablets are always taken in the middle of a meal. If side-effects are still experienced, the patient is advised to reduce the dose to that previously found to be acceptable. The drug can then be cautiously increased at less frequent intervals. Using this scheme the patient can be titrated up to very high doses, but usually a total daily dose of 5 to 10 mg is sufficient. In amenorrhoeic women, gonadotrophin pulsatility and menstruation usually return rapidly (Figure 7.4).

Bromocriptine is effective in virtually all cases of hyperprolactinaemia, although there are occasional cases of resistance. Bromocriptine is now the treatment of choice to suppress puerperal lactation, and has replaced all other medical treatment because it is so safe. The patient can be immediately started on a full dose of 2.5 mg twice daily if started within 48 h of delivery, as the drug is surprisingly free of side-effects when administered puerperally. A course of 10 to 14 days is usually sufficient.

Over the last 10 years extensive use of bromocriptine to treat infertility in countries throughout the world has failed to show any evidence of teratogenicity. However, it is still considered wise in most centres to advise women to stop bromocriptine therapy as soon as conception is confirmed, by the use of a sensitive pregnancy test a few days after a missed menstruation. There is evidence that pituitary macroadenomas in both sexes shrink in size on bromocriptine therapy, occasionally within a matter of days.

Bromocriptine is difficult to manufacture because a tripeptide moiety has to be linked to the basic ergot nucleus. Early attempts to use the ergot nucleus alone, as in lergotrile, were confounded when lergotrile was found to be hepatotoxic. Lisuride is similar in structure, and also has pronounced anti-serotonin activity;

Figure 7.4: Changes in LH (●——●) and FSH (○——○) Pulsatility in a Hyperprolactinaemic Patient Starting Treatment with Bromocriptine. (Taken from Moult *et al.* (1981), *Clinical Endocrinology, 16*, 153-62; reproduced by permission of the authors, and the Editors of *Clinical Endocrinology*.)

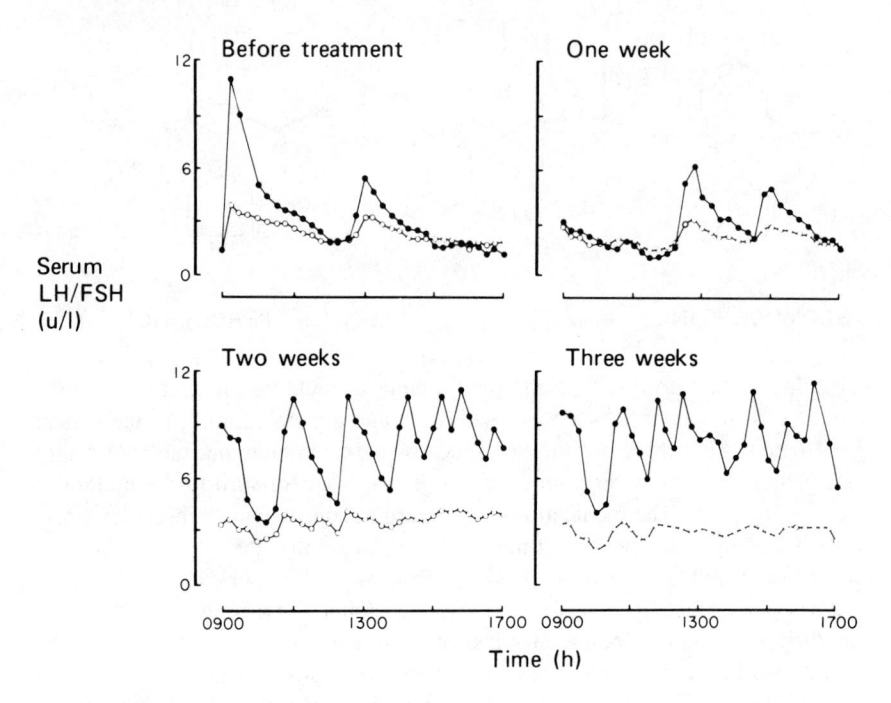

it has been in use for many years in Eastern Europe as an anti-migraine drug. In the treatment of hyperprolactinaemia, clinical trials have demonstrated a slightly higher incidence of side-effects than is seen with bromocriptine, and the drug has a shorter duration of action. By contrast, the new ergoline pergolide can usually be administered on a once-daily basis, and this may well represent a significant advance. In addition, there are occasional patients who respond to one drug rather than another in terms of freedom from side-effects, such that a choice of dopamine receptor agonists will be therapeutically useful. However, at the time of writing, only bromocriptine is generally available, and it is certainly the drug of which most experience has been obtained.

Further Reading

Auer, L.M., Leb, G., Tscherne, G., Urdl, W. and Walter, G.F. (1985) *Prolactinomas: an Interdisciplinary Approach*, De Gruyter, Berlin

Besser, G.H. (1983) 'Hyperprolactinaemia: Effects on Reproductive Function in Humans', in R.L. Norman (ed.), *Neuroendocrine Aspects of Reproduction*, pp. 345-57, Academic Press, New York

Franks, S. and Jacobs, H.S. (1983) 'Hyperprolactinaemia', *Clinics in Endocrinology and Metabolism, 12*, 641-68

Grossman, A. and Besser, G.M. (1985) 'Regular Review: Prolactinomas', *British Medical Journal*, *290*, 182–4
Leong, D.M., Frawley, L.S. and Neill, J.D. (1981) 'Neuroendocrine Control of Prolactin Secretion', *Annual Review of Physiology*, *43*, 109–27
Nabarro, J.D.N. (1982) 'Pituitary prolactinomas', *Clinical Endocrinology*, *17*, 129–55
Nicoll, C.S. (1980) 'Prolactin' (Symposium), *Federation Proceedings*, *39*, 2561–98
Vance, M.L., Evans, W.S. and Thorner, M.O. (1984) 'Bromocriptine', *Annals of Internal Medicine*, *100*, 78–91
Vogt, J.L. (1978) 'Control of Hormone Release during Lactation', *Clinics in Obstetrics and Gynaecology*, *5*, 435–56

8 GROWTH HORMONE, SOMATOSTATIN AND GROWTH HORMONE RELEASING HORMONE

Introduction

Interest in gigantism and acromegaly has spanned the centuries. A portrait of the father-in-law of Tutankhamun in approximately 1365 BC illustrates some of the features of acromegaly, and Old Testament writings have many reports of giants. It was not, however, until the late eighteenth century that Saucerette described a subject with features suggestive of acromegaly. Many reports appeared throughout the nineteenth century. In 1857 Chalk described dislocation of the lower jaw from an enlarged tongue associated with acromegaly, and seven years later Verga published the first post-mortem report of an acromegalic, describing the histology of a pituitary tumour; in 1886 Pierre Marie coined the term 'acromegaly'. The following year Minkowski noted the association of acromegaly with a pituitary tumour. The recognition of the particular connection with an eosinophil adenoma came in 1900. An early attempt at surgical treatment of acromegaly was made in 1893, and Cushing in 1912 and Schloffer in 1916 both operated on pituitary tumours by the nasal route.

When animal experimentation on growth first started, the only criterion for the demonstration of an effect was a change in body weight. In 1909, hypophysectomy was shown to cause dwarfism in a growing animal. Experimental gigantism was produced by Li and Evans in rats treated with extracts of anterior lobes, the animals developing to about twice the size of a normal adult. Another spectacular demonstration of the effect of pituitary extracts on growth was made by Evans and his co-workers in dachshunds. The picture of these animals has become very familiar as it is reproduced in many texts. This group also isolated bovine growth hormone. They first prepared alkaline extracts and subsequently an acetone powder, finally purifying the material in 1944. In 1957 Roben developed a method for the extraction of human growth hormone from pituitaries. Li and Dixon described the structure of human growth hormone (GH) and synthesised it in 1971.

Human growth hormone is a single-chain polypeptide containing 191 amino acids and has a molecular weight of around 22 000; the molecule has two disulphide bridges. On the basis of its sequence, growth hormone may be regarded as one of a family of peptides with related structures, including growth hormone, prolactin and human placental lactogen. Growth hormone isolated from the human pituitary resembles that from other species, but there are other considerable differences in primary structure, with ovine GH differing by approximately 70 residues from human GH. None of the other molecules is active in man. Any child deficient in the hormone cannot therefore be treated with preparations from any other species, and only extracts from human tissue can be used. Growth hormone is the most abundant peptide in the pituitary gland, with approximately 5 mg of growth hormone per gland, but the content does not change greatly with age. Growth hormone circulates in different forms in man. Analyses have shown that two species are present in the blood: 'big growth hormone' (which is twice the size of pituitary growth hormone), as well as one of the same molecular size as growth hormone. It also seems that a fragment of growth hormone may be responsible for some of the diabetogenic activity of the hormone. There are some problems associated with the measurement of growth hormone in plasma, since some bioassays may yield values up to one hundred times those obtained in radioimmunoassay. However, there is good agreement between the results of immunoassay and radioreceptor assays. Binding preparations for such assays may be obtained from a number of sources including liver and lymphocyte preparations.

Control of Hormone Secretion

As discussed in Chapter 3, release of growth hormone, like that of other anterior pituitary hormones, is controlled by a releasing factor but is also under the control of an inhibitory hormone, somatostatin. Again in common with other anterior pituitary hormones, such as ACTH, growth hormone secretion is episodic. Resting concentrations of growth hormone, determined by radioimmunoassay in the human adult, are usually less than 1 ng/ml (2 mU/litre). Striking variations are seen, with peaks of up to 20–40 ng/ml, which are particularly seen during non-dreaming slow-wave sleep at night. The hormone is rapidly cleared from the plasma, with a half-life of about 20–30 min. The basal concentrations are similar in the young and the adult so that it might appear that circulating growth hormone is not increased during puberty, the period of greatest growth. However, the bursts of growth hormone are of greater amplitude in the adolescent, so that the total growth-hormone secretion is greater. It has been calculated that in prepubertal children the mean 24-hour secretion rate is 91 μg, in adolescents 690 μg, and in young adults 35 μg. It then declines in later life.

On the basis of lesions and electrical stimulation performed in a number of animals including rat and monkey, it appears that the ventromedial nucleus (VMN) and particularly the adjoining arcuate nucleus are the final pathway for the integration of factors influencing the secretion of growth hormone. The VMN-basal hypothalamic pathway is the origin of the pulsatile pattern of stimulatory influences, whereas the preoptic basal hypothalamic pathways inhibit growth hormone secretion. Certain extrahypothalamic areas of the brain may also influence growth hormone secretion, as, for example, the hippocampus, amygdala and reticular formation, all of which have connections with the arcuate region of the hypothalamus. Growth hormone secretion is modified by three types of input: central nervous system inputs, metabolic influences and hormonal effects.

Central Nervous System Inputs

Extrahypothalamic structures exert a marked effect on growth hormone release. This is exemplified by the changes seen following sleep, stress and exercise. The

Figure 8.1: Typical 24 h Profile of Serum Growth Hormone in a Normal Subject

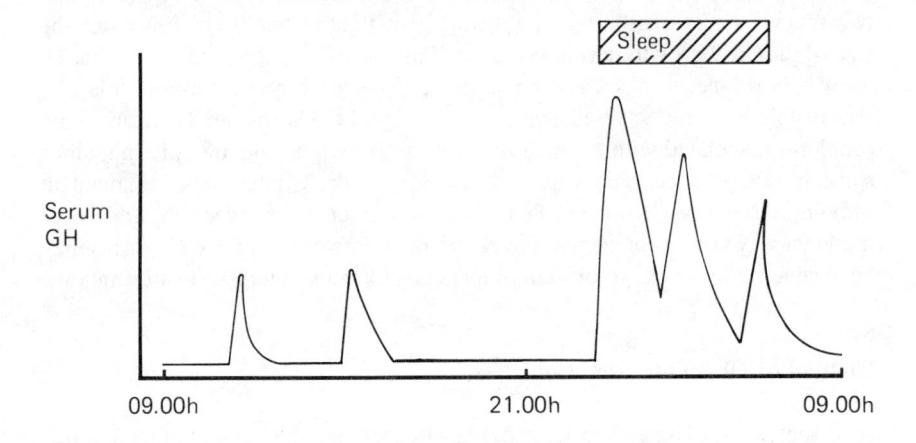

most marked changes are seen following the onset of sleep, so that it is possible that there is some truth in the old-wives' tale that one grows while one is asleep. Growth hormone secretion is temporally related to the beginning of period III or IV of sleep, i.e. slow-wave sleep. Up to 40 per cent of the total daily secretion may occur during this period of 1–2 hours (Figure 8.1). Growth hormone secretion nearly always corresponds to the period of deep sleep even if the onset of sleep is delayed or the sleep-wake cycle is reversed. If sleep is disturbed, then a second secretory peak may be seen.

Growth hormone, in common with ACTH, prolactin and vasopressin, is released in response to a number of stressful stimuli, including surgery. It is particularly stimulated by heavy exercise; psychological stress may produce similar circulating concentrations. In certain circumstances prolonged stress may apparently suppress growth hormone release. Thus children with gross emotional deprivation show secondary growth failure. One such example is said to be James Barrie, who suffered from maternal deprivation in his childhood and was less than 5 feet tall. Indeed, like his creation, Peter Pan, he never grew up. Many mechanisms may underly this response to stress, including metabolic and hormonal changes as described below. More recent studies have suggested that some emotionally deprived children have a disturbed sleep pattern such that slow-wave sleep occupies a smaller proportion of total sleep time.

Metabolic Influences

Metabolic products from the three major groups of foodstuffs, carbohydrates, proteins and fats, all affect growth hormone release. Glucose suppresses GH release, but there is a rebound of GH release in response to this suppression three to four hours after a meal. Insulin, which lowers blood glucose, has a profound effect on growth hormone release. The effect is probably mediated through glucose-sensitive receptors which lie in the lateral hypothalamus. Studies have shown that it is not the absolute concentration which is effective in GH secretion, but rather the change in concentration so that rising or falling glucose concentrations are the most effective stimuli. The effect on growth hormone secretion produced by physiological changes in blood glucose is relatively insignificant compared with that of exercise, sleep and stress, so that control of glucose homeostasis is probably a relatively less important function of growth hormone. However, the glucose effect is used as the basis of several growth hormone function tests. In addition to glucose metabolism, growth hormone secretion is linked to protein turnover. Following ingestion of a high-protein meal, increases in circulating GH concentration are seen; these can be reproduced by the infusion of several amino acids, particularly arginine and ornithine. In conclusion, although this aspect has been relatively less studied, elevated concentrations of plasma free fatty acids suppress stimulated and basal growth hormone secretion.

Hormonal Influences

Growth hormone secretion is modulated by other hormones. The plasma concentrations following exercise or infusion of arginine are frequently higher in women than in men, as are the levels of spontaneous GH secretion. This is most probably related to the oestrogen concentrations, as postmenopausal women have similar growth hormone secretion rates to those seen in men; it may depend on oestrogen-induced changes in somatomedins. Androgens have relatively little effect on growth hormone secretion. In contrast, glucocorticoids, in amounts comparable to those released by the adrenal cortex in times of stress, result in suppressed growth hormone secretion. There is also evidence that growth hormone exerts negative feedback on its own release. Part of this is probably due to the stimulation of somatostatin release by GH; some studies have also demonstrated negative-feedback effects of the somatomedins on the pituitary and hypothalamus. Glucagon, L-dopa and dopamine also release growth hormone in man. Vasopressin is effective in pharmacological doses.

Growth hormone responses to clinical test stimuli are impaired in many hypothyroid patients. However, TRH, although ineffective in stimulating GH release in normal subjects, produces a response in acromegaly as well as in renal failure, hepatic failure and anorexia nervosa. This may be a consequence of the changes in somatomedin concentrations in these conditions. Serum GH is generally suppressed in obesity and elevated in gross weight loss, including anorexia nervosa.

Neurotransmitters

As indicated in Chapter 4, all available evidence points to the fact that the classic neurotransmitters noradrenaline, dopamine, serotonin and acetylcholine are involved in the regulation of growth hormone secretion. Studies using adrenergic agonists and antagonists have shown that α-adrenergic and dopaminergic stimulation increase growth hormone secretion whereas β-adrenergic stimulation leads to decreased hormone release. The effects of catecholamines on growth hormone secretion are mediated via the hypothalamus. The noradrenergic activation is well established and probably operates via the α_2-adrenoceptors (clonidine is a particularly good stimulating drug);cholinergic antagonists block GH responses to many stimuli, probably by increasing somatostatin. Serotonin, histamine, GABA and the enkephalins are also important neurotransmitters in the stimulated release of GH, but it remains unclear as to whether most of these operate through somatostatin or growth hormone releasing hormone.

Action of Growth Hormone

As is implicit in the name, the main action of the hormone is to promote growth, characteristically in the immature subject. The hormone is most effective between birth and puberty. Even though the fetal animal appears to secrete marked amounts of hormone, it is not necessary for fetal growth. In the young animal before fusion of the epiphyses, the hormone stimulates chondrogenesis, allowing growth of the long bones. Prolonged administration of growth hormone to the young results in gigantism: not only is there extension of the long bones, but all the tissues grow in size to keep pace with the metabolic requirements. In the adult, when the epiphyses are fused, there is obviously no growth of the long bones; instead there is thickening of certain bones and of soft tissues. Growth hormone exerts an influence on the metabolic processes in probably all the tissues of the organism. This, together with the fact that the response to growth hormone is not seen immediately, that the hormone exhibits species-specificity, and that hypophysectomy results in the removal of the effects of many hormones, makes GH a particularly difficult hormone to study.

Effect of Growth Hormone on Cartilage

Extension of the long bones occurs through widening of the cartilaginous epiphysial plates and deposition of the bone matrix. Growth hormone stimulates this process through an action on chondrogenesis and osteogenesis. The first major action of growth hormone on cartilage was revealed by the reduced incorporation of radioactive sulphate into the tissue when the pituitary was removed. This probably resulted from a fall in chondroitin sulphate synthesis. Since then it has been shown that growth hormone affects other processes including the incorporation of amino acids into mucopolysaccharide complexes, and of uridine and thymidine into RNA and DNA, respectively, and also the conversion of proline to hydroxyproline. It is generally accepted that these effects on cartilage are *not* produced by growth hormone directly, but by somatomedins.

Somatomedins

Even though the growth-promoting effects of GH are easy to demonstrate *in vivo*, few investigators were originally able to show an effect on cell proliferation *in vitro*. However, in 1957, Salmon and Daughaday made the important observation that whereas addition of growth hormone to cartilage explants had little effect on the incorporation of $^{35}SO_4$ or tritiated thymidine, responses could be elicited by incubating the cartilage with serum from normal rats. The factor thus demonstrated to be present in plasma was originally named 'sulphation factor' and was later redesignated somatomedin. Subsequent work revealed that the factor comprised three somatomedins, A, B and C, of molecular weight 6000–9000. The idea of growth-promoting factors in serum is not a new one, as serum is regularly used in cell culture media. The chemical nature of serum-derived activity was shown in 1978 when insulin-like growth factor (IGF-I) was sequenced. A related peptide, IGF-II, has also been described, as has a factor necessary for cell proliferation — multiplication-stimulating activity (MSA). With clarification of the amino acid sequence of these various peptides, certain identities between pairs of them became obvious. For example, both IGFs are very similar to each other and to pro-insulin, and it is now accepted that IGF-I and somatomedin C are the same peptide. Somatomedin B is no longer thought to be a member of the original family as it lacks sulphation factor activity. Somatomedin A is very similar or even identical to somatomedin C, and IGF-II is non-GH-dependent and is related to MSA.

The role of somatomedins as mediators of the growth-promoting effects of growth hormone has only recently been definitely demonstrated, partly as a result of a shortage of pure peptides. Now, partially purified somatomedin has been used to demonstrate growth stimulation in the mouse. Infusion of IGF-I and IGF-II given via minipumps has been shown to cause a significant increase in tibial width and body weight in the hypophysectomised rat. *In vivo* purified somatomedins have an anabolic effect, stimulating thymidine uptake into DNA, DNA synthesis and mitosis in cells capable of proliferation. In addition to the growth-promoting activities, somatomedins possess remarkable insulin-like properties. In adipose tissue they stimulate lipid synthesis and glucose oxidation, inhibit the lipolytic activity of noradrenaline, and stimulate transport of amino acids and glucose across cell membranes of muscle and the synthesis of proteins. It appears that there are at least two types of receptor to account for these activities, a somatomedin receptor and one related to that for insulin.

In the circulation, somatomedins are bound to a carrier protein, which explains their long half-life in plasma and assures a continuous supply of the hormones to the target organs. They are the only peptide hormones to be protein bound. The principal source of the circulating somatomedins is primarily the liver, although other cells and organs may contribute. Many assays have been developed for somatomedins. Bioassays, radioreceptor assays, protein binding assays and radioimmunoassays have been developed, the bioassays depending on a number of factors including incorporation of ^{35}S-sulphate into the cartilage of hypophysectomised rats, conversion of ^{14}C-glucose into carbon dioxide in fat pads, and incorporation of tritiated thymidine into DNA.

These assays have demonstrated that different forms of somatomedin may predominate at different stages of life. In general, somatomedin C (IGF-I) increases gradually during childhood and then rises very rapidly during puberty before falling again to reach adult levels. Intra-uterine growth is independent of somatomedin C, and may require IGF-II. There is evidence that neuronal development requires a locally produced somatomedin *in utero*. Because of its long half-life there is no circadian rhythm of somatomedin C, but its level will fall with prolonged fasting.

Action of Growth Hormone on Protein Synthesis

Growth hormone has both anabolic and metabolic effects. The anabolic effects are related to growth promotion, enhanced formation of protein and nucleic acids, and the retention of other constituents of lean body mass, whereas the effects on fat and carbohydrate are metabolic effects supportive of anabolism and growth. As with other peptide hormones, the first step in its action is binding to specific receptors on the plasma membrane. Specific binding sites have been prepared from membrane fractions obtained from homogenates of liver from rabbits or rats. Studies on the binding sites have also been performed on lymphocyte preparations, and this phenomenon has been utilised in a novel GH bioassay. Growth hormone could affect protein synthesis at any one of a number of sites. It could stimulate the entry of amino acids into the cell and hence their availability for increased incorporation into protein. It could also act at the nuclear level in the transcription of new mRNA, or it could influence the rate at which ribosomes translate mRNA. Studies monitoring the uptake of radioactive-labelled amino acids have revealed that growth hormone does indeed stimulate amino acid uptake. Using actinomycin D (which blocks transcription), and puromicin (which blocks translation), it is possible to distinguish between nuclear and non-nuclear events. This techinque revealed that the rapid effect of growth hormone on protein synthesis is on the translational process. In the longer term, however, growth hormone administration does result in increased production of ribosomal RNA. The positive nitrogen balance is accompanied by retention of sodium, potassium, magnesium and chloride. It is not clearly established how growth hormone produces its effect at the ribosomal level, but it has been suggested that this could be related to a fall in the cyclic AMP concentration.

Action of Growth Hormone on Carbohydrate Metabolism

Chronic growth hormone administration to a normal animal has a diabetogenic effect. It produces an increase in the fasting blood glucose concentration, resulting in part from increased glucose output from the liver and in part from inhibition of the action of insulin on entry of glucose into tissues. There is also an increase in the glycogen content in the liver, which in turn could lead to an increase in blood glucose. There has been considerable debate as to the mechanism underlying the decreased sensitivity to insulin, but it may in part be due to reduction of glucose phosphorylation in the tissues. In normal subjects with a predisposition to diabetes mellitus, GH produces an increased hyperglycaemic response with acidosis. Recent studies have suggested that this predisposition is genetically linked. In contrast to this effect in normal animals, growth hormone when injected into an untreated hypophysectomised animal produces a prompt hypoglycaemia which is especially noticeable in the young animal. There is also a fall in liver and muscle glycogen. This insulin-like effect is only seen in response to a single injection of growth hormone and is not seen after second and subsequent injections are given. That this effect is due to the absence of growth hormone rather than ACTH can be demonstrated by the observation that treatment with glucocorticoid does not influence the response. This insulin-like activity of growth hormone has probably little effect on the normal regulation of carbohydrate metabolism.

Action of Growth Hormone on Lipid Metabolism

Growth hormone increases the concentration of free fatty acids in the plasma of both man and animals, and inhibits fat synthesis. This occurs by a direct effect not dependent on somatomedin. It has been suggested that growth hormone may not itself initiate lipolysis, but is required for the lipolytic activity of other agents. The fact that free fatty acid concentrations do not accompany the growth hormone spurts seen during sleep has been taken as evidence that growth hormone plays little role in lipid metabolism under normal circumstances.

Somatostatin

In searching for the elusive growth hormone releasing hormone (GHRH), Brazeau and colleagues at the Salk Institute in La Jolla, California, came across a hypothalamic peptide in 1973 that *inhibited* growth hormone release. The existence of such a factor had been predicted by Krulich and McCann in 1968. It was found that this cyclic 14-residue peptide (Figure 8.2) was extremely potent in both cyclic and linear forms in inhibiting growth hormone release *in vitro* and *in vivo* in the rat. Early work suggested that somatostatin caused multiple petechial haemorrhages in certain primates when administered in high doses. However, this now appears to be species-specific, as extensive short-term studies have demonstrated the safety of somatostatin administration in man. It has been found that many other hormones and activities are inhibited by somatostatin, including the release of TSH and, under certain circumstances, prolactin and ACTH. Because of this it was at one time thought that somatostatin was a generalised non-specific 'inhibitor', suppressing the function of all biological tissues. However, it is now realised that the actions of somatostatin are indeed specific, and are mediated through its own receptors which involve cyclic AMP and calcium influx.

Figure 8.2: Structural Formula of Somatostatin

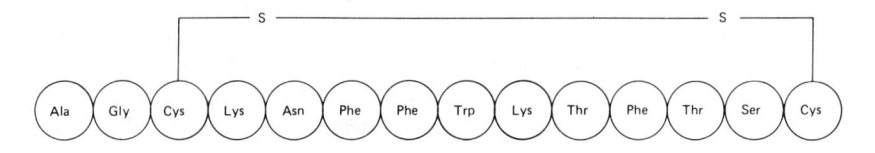

Ala — Gly — Cys — Lys — Asn — Phe — Phe — Trp — Lys — Thr — Phe — Thr — Ser — Cys

(S—S bridge between the two Cys residues)

Somatostatin has a widespread distribution throughout the central nervous system, autonomic nervous system and the gut. In the hypothalamus, somatostatin is concentrated in the anterior and periventricular areas with long curving axons sweeping down to terminate around the portal vessels in the median eminence. In the cerebral cortex, it may function as a classical neurotransmitter, and changes in CSF somatostatin have been reported in patients with Alzheimer's disease. In the gut, there is evidence for intestinal secretion into the gut lumen, and the pancreatic D cells in the islets contain somatostatin, probably acting in a paracrine role in modulating the nearby insulin and glucagon cells. Circulating somatostatin is probably derived from the gut and pancreas, but whether the changes in levels following food stimuli are truly indicative of an endocrine function is currently unknown. The most recent data suggest that gut somatostatin functions as an enterogastrone to inhibit stomach secretion in response to fat reaching the duodenum.

In the rat, stress induces a fall in growth hormone release and there is some evidence that this is principally due to the release of somatostatin. Somatostatin release is also stimulated by dopaminergic agents and possibly noradrenaline, and is modulated in a more complex function by opioid peptides. It should be noted that in the rat, but not in man, hypoglycaemia is suppressive of growth hormone. Nevertheless, the functional importance of somatostatin remains uncertain. Most studies, using either injected somatostatin antiserum or stalk-sectioned animals, have suggested that somatostatin plays a minor modulatory role as compared with GHRH. Most spontaneous GH secretory peaks appear to be a consequence of an increase in GHRH release rather than a fall in somatostatin. However, it is likely that at least part of the feedback effect of the somatomedins is medicated through somatostatin release, and it has been suggested that much of the variability of the response of serum GH to exogenous GHRH in man is due to changes in endogenous somatostatin. It has also been postulated that a defect in hypothalamic somatostatin is primary in initiating acromegaly, although there is little good evidence for this. Somatostatin levels in the CSF remain unaltered in this condition, but hypothalamic levels have not, as yet, been assessed.

More recently, a putative 28-residue precursor of somatostatin has been described in which the N-terminus of somatostatin-14 is extended. It is at least as potent as somatostatin-14. As somatostatin-14 and 28 are apparently released from the hypothalamus in a constant ratio of approximately 2 : 1 it seems probable that somatostatin-28 is a hormone in its own right, and that both peptides are derived from a common precursor.

Therapeutically, somatostatin has been used to treat pancreatitis, gastrointestinal haemorrhage and hormone-secreting tumours of islet cells. Research has been hampered by the absence of an orally active preparation and by the short half-life of somatostatin. An 8-residue analogue recently developed has shown considerable promise in the treatment of acromegaly. Although this analogue still has to be given parenterally, it is considerably longer acting than native somatostatin-14. It is likely that somatostatin analogues will eventually play a major role in the treatment of acromegaly.

GHRH

One of the most exciting discoveries in neuroendocrinology over the last five years has been the nature of the structure of human GHRH. For many years it has been known that certain human tumours can ectopically produce a GHRH, and such patients may indeed present with acromegaly. In 1982, Michael Thorner, working in Virginia, submitted an acromegalic patient to trans-sphenoidal hypophysectomy, but was surprised to be told that no tumour could be located. Histologically, in place of tumour tissue there was somatotroph hyperplasia. A subsequent search revealed a pancreatic carcinoid tumour, and it was postulated that this tumour was secreting a GHRH that stimulated the pituitary somatotrophs. Whereas the extraction of at least half a million ovine or porcine hypothalami had failed to produce the structure of GHRH, this sequence was rapidly deduced by extraction of this human pancreatic tumour by Wylie Vale and his colleagues. This revealed a surprisingly large peptide of 40 amino acids, which was related to the glucagon-cholecystokinin family of peptides. Simultaneously, Roger Guillemin and his colleagues at the Salk Institute extracted GH releasing factors from a pancreatic tumour removed from a patient in Lyons, France. The majority of biological activity was found to be associated with a peptide identical to that isolated by Vale (hpGRF 1–40). There were also significant amounts of an amidated C-terminal extended form (hpGRF-1–44), and minor amounts of the shortened analogue hpGRF 1–37. Studies in man have demonstrated that both the (1–40) and (1–44) analogues are potent stimulators of growth hormone release, and it seems highly probable that hypothalamic GHRH is highly similar or identical to either or both peptides.

Immunostaining has revealed that primate GHRH is synthesised in the area homologous to the arcuate nucleus in the rat. Interestingly enough, rat GHRH is relatively dissimilar to hpGRF. It contains 43 amino acids, and differs in approximately 30 per cent of its residues. *In vitro*, hpGRF 1–40 and 1–44 stimulate rat somatotrophs to release growth hormone, and similar results are obtained with human acromegalic cells in culture. The response is mediated via cyclic AMP and there is non-competitive antagonism with somatostatin.

Studies in normal humans have shown that growth hormone release is highly variable after any of the GHRH analogues, including the potent derivative hpGRF (1–29) amide. This may be due to endogenous release of somatostatin. In patients with large hypothalamic tumours, such as craniopharyngiomas and germinomas, hypoglycaemia-stimulated release of growth hormone may be absent while responsiveness remains to exogenous GHRH analogues. This suggests that such patients are deficient in the production or release of endogenous GHRH or, in the case of large pituitary tumours, in the accessibility of endogenous GHRH to somatotrophs via the portal vasculature. Since GHRH is required for growth hormone synthesis, as well as the stimulation of the readily releasable pool, long-term deficiency of endogenous GHRH will eventually lead to failure of the somatotrophs to respond to exogenous GHRH acutely. Most recently, the 'growth hormone deficiency' seen after irradiation of the hypothalamo-pituitary axis has

100 *Growth Hormone, Somatostatin and GHRH*

Figure 8.3: Serum GH Responses to GHRH (1-40) Given in a Dose of 200 μg i.v. in Five Children with Isolated GH Deficiency in whom Insulin-induced Hypoglycaemia Induced No Rise in Serum GH. Four of these five children showed a clear response to GHRH. (A. Grossman, M.O. Savage and G.M. Besser, unpublished observations.)

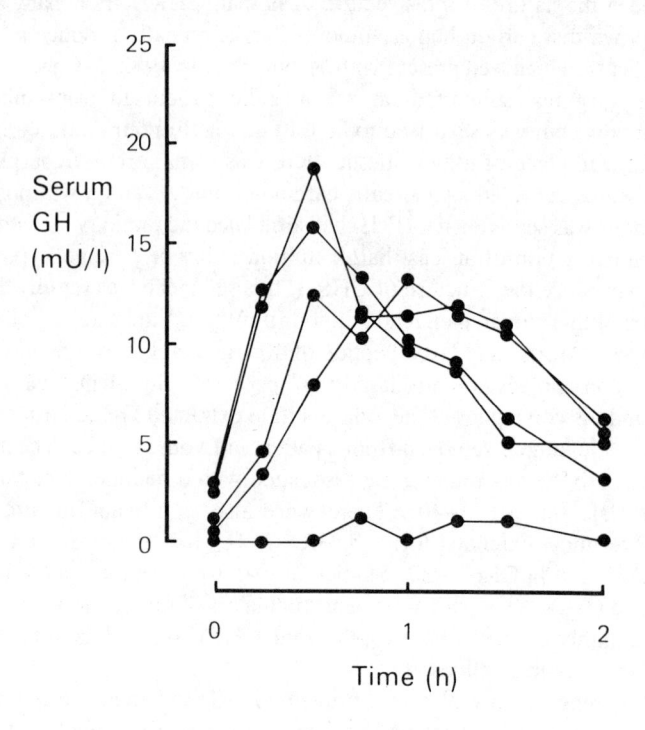

been shown to be secondary to changes in endogenous GHRH. Furthermore, it now appears that many children with idiopathic growth hormone deficiency or panhypopituitarism can respond to exogenous GHRH with a rise in serum growth hormone and somatomedin (Figure 8.3). It has long been known that many such children do indeed have somatotrophs present in the pituitary, and thus are not deficient in growth hormone *per se*. Ongoing studies into long-term subcutaneous or intranasal administration of GHRH analogues indicate that this may well be an acceptable form of therapy in such children.

Clinical Syndromes

Acromegaly and Gigantism

Oversecretion of growth hormone results in gigantism before the epiphyses have fused, and acromegaly thereafter. In acromegaly there is progressive enlargement of the soft tissues of the hands and feet, and further growth of certain of the bones of the skull, particularly the lower jaw (Table 8.1). The fingers become broad and spatulate, the supraorbital ridges enlarge and the characteristic facies appears, most notably the prognathism. Other symptoms of acromegaly include increased perspiration in both sexes and hirsuties/acne/seborrhoea in women. On examination, additional features usually include hypertension, a multinodular goitre in one-third of cases, and a thoracic kyphosis in long-standing cases. Many patients are diagnosed while being assessed for other unrelated conditions, or come to the attention of a physician for treatment of related hypertension or hyperglycaemia. The condition is usually so insidious that the change in facies and body habitus goes unnoticed by the patient and his family, and may only be noted by a medical attendant who has never or only rarely seen the patient before. It is generally concluded that acromegaly has a prevalence of 40 cases per million, with an incidence of three new cases per million. It is possible that the apparent rarity of the condition is at least in part a reflection of this phenomenon, and that its true prevalence is much higher than commonly realised. Almost invariably the condition is caused by a growth hormone-secreting pituitary adenoma, usually an eosinophil or chromophobe adenoma. Local pressure affects (headache, field defects) are not uncommon, and may be the mode of presentation. Hypopituitarism is also seen, particularly hypogonadism, although rarely more severe pituitary destruction may take place.

Biochemically, the characteristic feature is an elevation of serum growth hormone which, though pulsatile and occasionally highly variable, is never undetectable and does not peak during sleep. Diagnostically, if, in a series of four or more blood samples, growth hormone never becomes undetectable (< 0.5 ng/ml), acromegaly should be considered. The standard diagnostic test is the failure of suppression of growth hormone during a standard glucose tolerance test (Chapter 14). Other biochemical changes noted in such patients are an elevated serum phosphate, hypercalcaemia (5-10 per cent) and hypercalciuria (70 per cent), glucose intolerance (30 per cent) or frank diabetes mellitus (10 per cent), and hyperprolactinaemia in about one-third of patients. The latter may be due to tumour disruption of delivery of dopamine to the lactotrophs, a mixed tumour of prolactin and growth hormone cells, or on rare occasions a homogeneous tumour of cells secreting both prolactin and growth hormone. Recent studies on vitamin D metabolism have demonstrated that growth hormone stimulates the renal enzyme 1α-hydroxylase, thus possibly explaining the hypercalciuria of acromegaly. However, some patients do have co-existent primary hyperparathyroidism and thus features of the syndrome of the multiple endocrine adenomatosis type I. Currently the hypertension is unexplained, although there appears to be an increase in total body sodium.

An abnormal pituitary fossa is visible radiologically in over 90 per cent of patients, possibly reflecting the long natural history of the disease. Suprasellar extensions are not uncommon.

It has been clearly shown that survival is shortened in patients with acromegaly, and thus treatment is mandatory in all but the oldest patients or those with minimal disease. Trans-sphenoidal surgery is most often employed and can be curative (c. 80 per cent) in patients with small tumours (microadenomas). However, as has been noted, the majority of patients have macroadenomas and in such patients

Table 8.1: Clinical and Biochemical Features of Acromegaly

Symptoms
   Sweating
   Increase in shoe and/or glove size
   Change in ring size
   Malocclusion of teeth
   Carpal tunnel syndrome
   Female: amenorrhoea/hirsuties
   Male: poor libido/erectile failure

Signs
   Distortion of facial features, including prognathism
   Osteoarthrosis
   Multinodular goitre
   Dorsal kyphosis
   Spatulate hands
   Increased skin thickness
   Female: hirsuties/acne
   Male: hypogonadism
   Hypertension

N.B. There may be additional features associated with a large pituitary tumour, e.g. headache, visual field defects and hypopituitarism

Biochemistry
   Glucose tolerance test: serum growth hormone fails to suppress and may rise paradoxically
   TRH test: serum growth hormone rises c. 80%
   LHRH test: serum growth hormone rises c. 10%
   CRF test: no rise in serum growth hormone ⎫ No distinction between
   GHRH test: variable rise in serum growth hormone ⎭ normals and acromegalics
   Serum prolactin: elevated basally in c. 30%
   Serum calcium: elevated in c. 10%; ? coexistent with hyperparathyroidism
   Hypercalciuria: present in 70%
   Serum phosphate: elevated
   Sex hormone binding globulin (SHBG): depressed in the female
   Thyroid function tests ⎫
   Gonadal function tests   Abnormal with large
   Posterior pituitary function   space-occupying
   Adrenocortical function ⎭ lesion
   Diabetes mellitus: impaired tolerance in 30%; frankly abnormal in 10%

radiotherapy may be highly effective in lowering serum growth hormone levels over a period of years. Most experience has been gained with megavoltage external radiotherapy; at a total tumour dose of 4500 cGy serum growth hormone falls progressively year by year and is below 10 mU/litre in about 80 per cent of patients after 10 years. However, this is clearly a long time to wait for disease control. Fortunately, Liuzzi and co-workers first noted, in 1974, that the dopamine agonist bromocriptine lowers serum growth hormone in 60–70 per cent of patients with acromegaly, although really marked falls are only seen in 30 per cent. This effect is paradoxical in that dopaminergic agents *elevate* growth hormone in normal subjects. Other abnormalities of growth hormone release by neurotransmitters include a stimulation of release by GnRH (in 10 per cent) and TRH (in 80 per cent). These aberrant responses are not necessarily manifestations of abnormal tumour receptors, as similar responses have been reported in a patient with somatotroph hyperplasia secondary to ectopic GHRH secretion. Thus, bromocriptine may be used to lower growth hormone in certain responsive patients while awaiting the full effects of radiotherapy. Although large doses may be required (up to 60 mg/day) the majority of patients require 10–30 mg of bromocriptine a day. A reasonable management policy would be to assess bromocriptine responsiveness in all patients with acromegaly, and in those demonstrating a clear chemical and biochemical improvement, external radiotherapy can then be administered. In those patients relatively unresponsive to bromocriptine, especially when growth hormone levels are particularly high and the pituitary fossa is not too abnormal, trans-sphenoidal surgery is preferable. For larger tumours, or when growth hormone is not normalised by surgery, it should be followed by radiotherapy. Following radiotherapy, all patients require regular reassessment of pituitary function, and patients apparently cured by surgery will need observation for possible tumour recurrence.

The long-term outlook is good in treated patients, although it may take years for facial features to improve. A loss of excess sweating is an early clinical sign of amelioration. It is unclear as to whether there is a specific cardiomyopathy associated with acromegaly, and whether it improves with treatment of the underlying condition.

Pituitary giants should be treated similarly to patients with acromegaly: in these patients it is especially important to achieve rapid control of growth hormone secretion to prevent psychosocial disabilities associated with excessively tall stature. It has been suggested that certain tall adolescents may demonstrate a pathological growth hormone response to TRH, and occasionally even a failure of growth hormone suppression during a glucose tolerance test in the absence of clinical acromegaly. However, this interesting finding requires further confirmation.

Growth Hormone Deficiency

Deficiency of growth hormone in the adult produces no obvious clinical symptoms, but in the child results in failure of growth and dwarfism. Such children are symmetrically small (Figure 8.4). Tumours, particularly craniopharyngiomas, may be the cause of the condition when it is acquired after birth, particularly when it occurs in association with other hormone deficiencies. In the case of congenital GH deficiency, it is possible that minimal birth trauma a causative factor in some .

Rarely, there may be a genetic defect in GH synthesis. Although growth hormone secretion may be low from birth, it is generally not noted for many months. Laron dwarfism is a type of dwarfism, in which growth hormone concentrations are paradoxically high but plasma somatomedin is low. In some African pygmies growth hormone levels are normal whereas somatomedin concentrations are low. In Turner's syndrome the peripheral tissues of the body appear to be unable to respond to normal levels of somatomedin.

104 *Growth Hormone, Somatostatin and GHRH*

Figure 8.4: Features of a Child with Typical Idiopathic GH Deficiency (courtesy of Dr M.O. Savage)

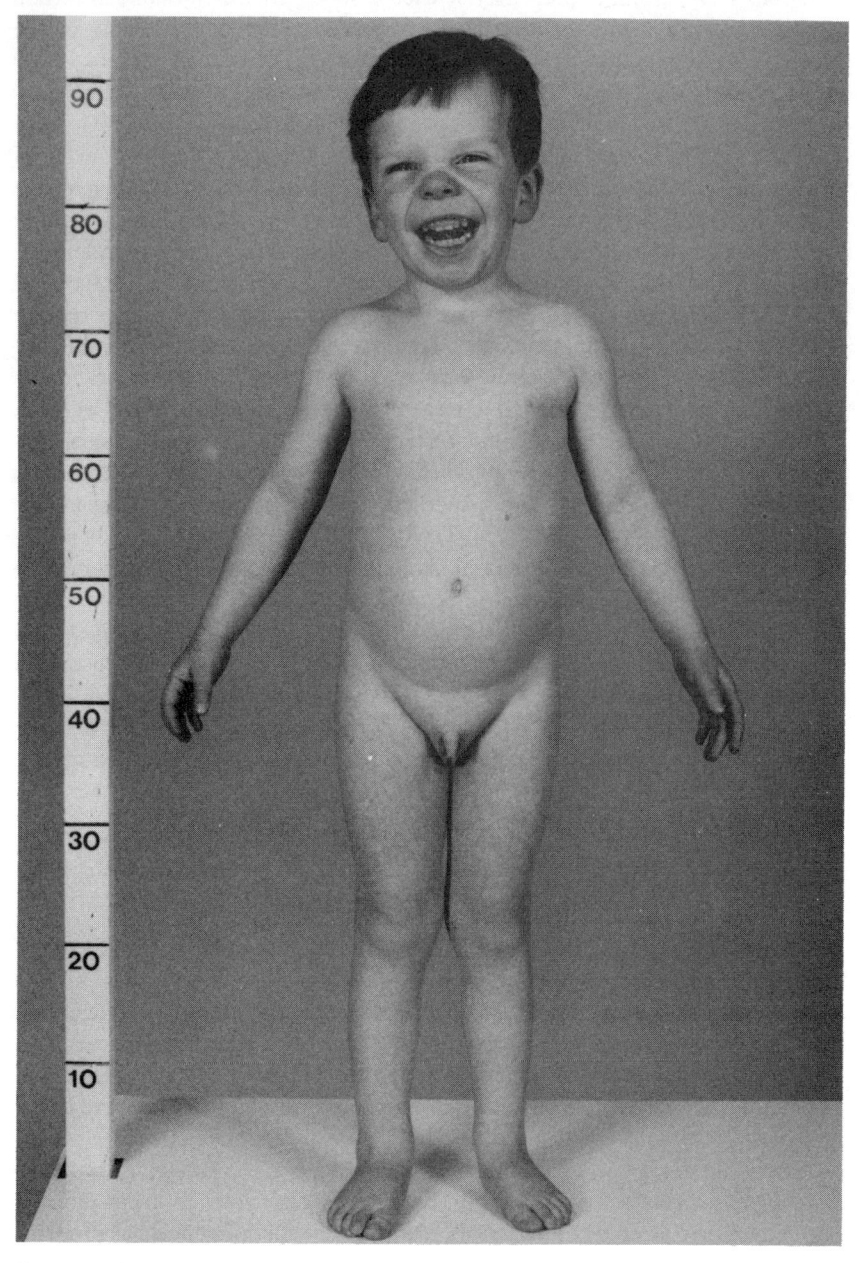

Over the years many provocative tests for growth hormone secretion have been employed. Unfortunately, the structural level at which these tests stimulate growth hormone release is unclear; the results are often variable, testing conditions poorly standardised, and occasional side-effects disrupting. L-dopa has been extensively used, but can cause nausea and vomiting. Arginine and 'Bovril' also stimulate growth hormone release through an unknown mechanism, and are little used nowadays. Exercise is also a potent stimulus to growth hormone but must be quite severe to be effective, and standardised values are not readily available. The most reliable stimulus is hypoglycaemia. In a standard insulin tolerance test (ITT) (see Chapter 14) a peak growth hormone response above 40 mU/ml is normal; values between 20 and 40 mU/ml are probably normal, and a peak below 20 mU/ml is abnormal. Occasionally, slightly subnormal results in prepubertal children may be normalised by treating such children with a short course of stilboestrol. However, the mechanism of this effect is unknown at present. In experienced hands the test is quite safe and reproducible. In children it is probably wise to use 0.1 U/kg of insulin rather than the adult dose of 0.15 U/kg. Recently, Laron and his colleagues have introduced the clonidine stimulation test for use in children and adolescents. This α_2-adrenoceptor agonist stimulates growth hormone release via the hypothalamus. The test is less well standardised than the ITT, with varying schedules of oral or parenteral administration, and is only a poor stimulus to growth hormone release in adults. Its principal side-effect is sedation. However, the UK Growth Hormone Committee have compared its use with the ITT in children of short stature and in the majority of cases there is concordance between the two tests.

The diagnosis of growth hormone deficiency in the child with short stature is not always straightforward. It is less difficult in patients with hypothalamic tumours in whom a fall in growth velocity is occasionally the first sign of incipient hypopituitarism. Other features consistent with the tumour are present, and usually a good response is seen with growth hormone therapy (Figure 8.5). In the child with isolated idiopathic growth hormone deficiency, a normal birth weight and length are seen, but deviation from the normal growth curve is seen progressively year by year. The child is usually excessively fat and has a retarded bone age in relation to its chronological age. Sometimes, the response to hypoglycaemia is diagnostic, with no growth hormone response. In the case of a partial response, a second different test is advisable. A deficient response to both tests is highly suggestive of growth hormone deficiency and, after a period of documented low growth velocity, growth hormone therapy can be started. In children with short stature and one or both tests normal, it is not usually advised that growth hormone can be given therapeutically. However, recent studies have suggested that even these children may benefit, and treatment is more often rejected due to limitation in supply rather than poor therapeutic expectations. Growth hormone has usually been extracted from cadaveric pituitaries, and has been given as a subcutaneous or intramuscular injection two or three times a week. However, owing to the discovery of cases of Jacob-Creutzfeldt disease with a prevalence of 1 in 1000 in patients treated with cadaveric GH (normal prevalence 1 in 10^6),

Figure 8.5: Typical Growth Chart of a Child with Growth Hormone Deficiency. Note the acceleration in growth when human growth hormone is given

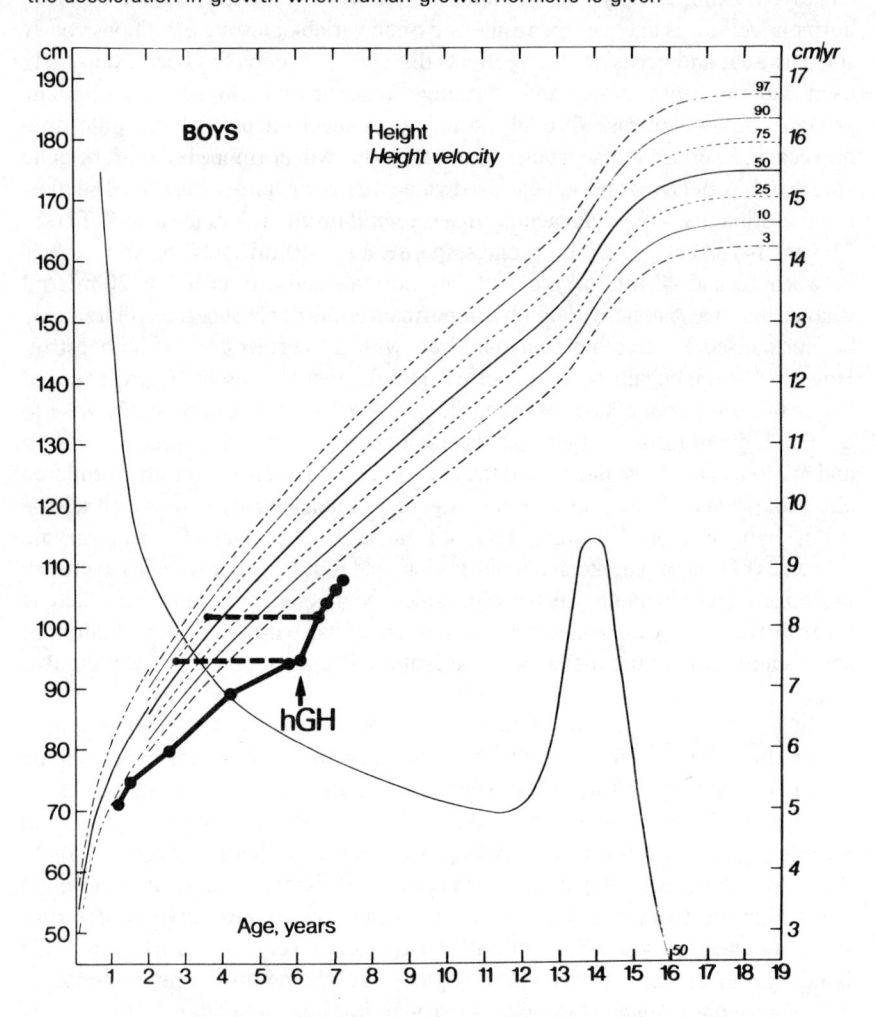

such treatment was stopped in most Western countries in early 1985. It is currently being replaced by biosynthetic GH. Growth must be assessed in special auxological centres, but rarely is the expected 'mid-parental' height achieved. It is possible that spreading the same weekly doses of growth hormone by daily injection will be more effective, or that biogenetically engineered analogues of GH or GHRH (see above) will be in greater supply and thus allow greater rates of growth. In panhypopituitary patients, sex hormone therapy will be required at around the time of puberty, although the fact that such treatment will lead to epiphyseal closure needs to be taken into account. It is evident that the diagnosis and treatment of short stature is currently far from satisfactory.

Further Reading

Besser, G.M. and Wass, J.A.H (1984) 'The Medical Management of Acromegaly', in Black, P.M., Zervas, N.T., Ridgway, E.C. and Martin, J.B. (eds), *Secretory Tumors of the Pituitary Gland*, pp. 155-68, Raven Press, New York

Laws, E.R., Randall, R. and Abboud, C.F. (1982) 'Pathophysiology of Acromegaly: Results in 140 Patients', in J.A. Givens (ed.), *Hormone-secreting Pituitary Tumors*, pp. 209-24, Year Book Medical Publishers, Chicago

Hall, K. and Sara, V.R. (1983) 'Growth and Somatomedins', *Vitamins and Hormones, 40*, 175-233

Tanner, J.M. (1981) *Control of Growth*, Churchill Livingstone, Edinburgh

Van Wyk, J.J. and Underwood, L.E. (1980) 'Growth Hormone, Somatomedins and Growth Failure', in D.T. Krieger and J.C. Hughes (eds), *Neuroendocrinology — a Hospital Practice Book*, pp. 229-309, Sinauer, Sunderland, Mass.

Wass, J.A.H. (1983) 'Growth Hormone Neuroregulation and the Clinical Relevance of Somatostatin', *Clinics in Endocrinology and Metabolism, 12*, 695-724

9 THE GONADOTROPHINS AND LUTEINISING HORMONE RELEASING HORMONE

Historical Introduction

It is not easy to identify the origins of research into the role of the anterior pituitary in influencing gonadal function. However, such a link had been suggested by the observation of Harvey Cushing that there was a reduction in the size of the gonads on hypophysectomy, and of Aschner, who noted persistent infantilism in hypophysectomised puppies. A further indication was provided by Long and Evans, who observed ovarian enlargement in rats treated with growth-promoting extracts. None the less, the first demonstration of a positive influence of the anterior lobe on the gonads was made independently in 1926 by Smith and by Zondek and Ascheim, who noted that daily implants of fresh anterior-lobe tissue induced rapid growth of the ovary and uterus. Considerable confirmatory data were produced over the next five years. The first evidence that there were two gonadotrophins came from the finding by Ascheim and Zondek that the urine of pregnant women contained a principle with luteinising activity whereas the urine of post-menopausal women produced predominantly a follicle-stimulating response. It was, however, a matter of some debate as to whether the pituitary produced two active components or whether the material found in the urine of pregnant women was actually of placental origin. The first report of a separation of the two activities from extracts of pituitary came in 1931, but acceptance of the two-hormone concept was not universal for many years. At one point it was suggested that interstitial cell stimulating hormone (ICSH) was an additional independent gonadotrophin in the male, although it was later shown to be identical with luteinising hormone (LH). Relatively pure preparations of LH and follicle stimulating hormone (FSH) were made in the 1940s by Li and Evans, but at this time chemical purification of these hormones presented considerable problems. It is now accepted that the gonadotrophins LH, FSH and human chorionic gonadotrophin (HCG) are all glycoprotein hormones composed of two subunits, a β-subunit, which is hormone specific, and an α-subunit, which is common to these three hormones as well as to TSH. The biological specificity is conferred by the β-chains so that a hybrid formed, for example, between the subunit of TSH and the β-subunit of LH would possess the biological characteristics of native LH. The subunits exert no biological activity. Human chorionic gonadotrophin is synthesised in the placenta and has similar biological properties to those of LH. The amino acid composition of LH and FSH varies considerably. LH is relatively conserved across species, suggesting that the primary structure is similar, but the molecular weight varies from 26 000 in man to 55 400 in horse, probably due to differing amounts of attached sugar residues. The remainder of this section will be concerned primarily with the pituitary gonadotrophins.

Control of Secretion

Both FSH and LH are synthesised and stored in cells of the anterior pituitary, their secretion being under the control both of hypothalamic releasing hormone and of the gonadal steroids. Regulation of secretion is by a rather complex interaction of neural and hormonal components. The maintenance of normal reproductive function in both the male and the female depends on the existence of a delicately balanced relationship between the hypothalamus, the anterior pituitary and the gonads. Although the pituitary hormones involved are the same in both sexes, the system in the male is geared to the continuous production of spermatozoa, whereas in the female a cyclical process operates to produce an ovum at a particular frequency depending on the species.

Most evidence points to the presence of just one hypothalamic hormone stimulating the secretion of both LH and FSH, although this is not universally accepted. This hypothalamic regulator is variously termed luteinising hormone releasing hormone (LHRH), gonadotrophin releasing hormone (GnRH) or LH/FSH-RH. However, the question as to the occurrence of a separate FSH releasing hormone remains to be answered.

Both LH and FSH are released in episodic pulses seen at a frequency of one every one or two hours. This episodic release is controlled from the hypothalamus and higher centres: it is suggested that progesterone principally lowers the rate of pulses of LHRH and oestrogen augments the response to LHRH. Centrally acting drugs such as phenobarbitone and opiates, as well as hypothalamic lesions, abolish the pulsatile pattern. Thus the pulsatile release of gonadotrophins is thought to be secondary to the phasic discharge of LHRH from nerves terminating in the median eminence. These neurones are in turn modulated by a variety of hypothalamic neuroamines and neuropeptides. The secretion of LH and FSH is normally inhibited by elevated plasma concentrations of the gonadal steroids (i.e. negative feedback). Oestrogens are particularly potent inhibitors of LH and FSH release, LH being more sensitive to this feedback inhibition than FSH. The inhibitory effect of steroids is illustrated by the observation that gonadectomy results in an elevated concentration of the gonadotrophins and by their rise at the menopause. Oestrogen receptors are abundant both in the pituitary and in various brain areas, and most evidence suggests that both the pituitary and the hypothalamus are involved in the feedback inhibition exerted by the steroids; for example, direct injection of oestrogen into the third ventricle lowers the plasma LH in experimental preparations, and oestrogen has been shown to have direct effects on the anterior pituitary gland. Gonadotrophins may alter their own level of secretion by acting directly on the brain or pituitary, although the physiological significance of this short-loop feedback is questionable. A non-steroidal factor, inhibin, acting selectively on FSH, has been isolated. This substance is found in ovarian follicular fluid. In the female, just prior to ovulation the secretion of gonadotrophins is actually *stimulated* by the high plasma concentration of oestradiol (positive feedback) resulting in a mid-cycle surge of LH and FSH. For a positive feedback to be manifest, a critical level of oestrogen of approximately 300 pg/ml has to be achieved for a duration of 72 h. It appears that this positive feedback is exerted at the level of the pituitary.

The site of LHRH cell bodies in the central nervous system is rather controversial, some workers describing LHRH immunoreactive cells in the preoptic and suprachiasmatic regions and others finding cells in the arcuate nucleus. It is possible that fibres from both areas terminate in the median eminence. Recent studies in the rhesus monkey demonstrated that lesions of the arcuate nucleus led to cessation of the episodic release of LHRH and thus of LH release, and only when LHRH was infused in an episodic manner with a frequency of about one pulse per hour did the characteristic pattern of LH release resume. Less frequent administration of LHRH leads to a relative fall-off in pituitary response, but paradoxically so does more frequent administration, especially continuous infusion. This suggests that the hypothalamus must produce a pulse-frequency of LHRH release that has a well-defined upper limit to avoid down-regulation and desensitisation. It appears that pituitary LHRH receptors require the constant alternation of occupancy and non-occupancy to maintain their responsiveness, and this has clear therapeutic implications (see below).

For a number of years it was thought that dopamine was the major stimulus for LHRH release, and in fact dopamine does cause release of LHRH from hypothalamic synaptosomes. However, it now appears that dopamine has both stimulatory and inhibitory effects on hypothalamic LHRH release. There is much more evidence pointing towards adrenaline as a major influence on LHRH secretion, at least in the rat. Both adrenaline and noradrenaline are effective in releasing LHRH when injected into the third ventricle. Further evidence for the positive effects of noradrenaline on LH release comes from the observation that hypothalamic deafferentation, which causes a 60 per cent fall in the hypothalamic content of noradrenaline, blocks the pre-oestrus LH surge in the rat. In addition acetylcholine appears to be stimulatory to LHRH release, and there is evidence for an inhibitory effect of serotonin and melatonin. There is also evidence that prostaglandins play a role in LHRH release. Most of the studies described have concerned the hypothalamus, but other regions such as the amygdala, hippocampus and midbrain are also involved in gonadotrophin secretion. Unfortunately, studies in man are very few and there is little clear evidence for the neuroamine modulation of LHRH release, although endogenous opioids are undoubtedly important modulators of pulse frequency.

Release of Gonadotrophins during Development

As mentioned in Chapter 2, the human fetal hypothalamus synthesises LHRH at the 8th week of gestation, whereas gonadotrophins are produced by the 10th to 13th week. There are three phases of gonadotrophin secretion in the fetus. Initially, in early fetal life, circulating gonadotrophin concentrations are high as a result of unrestrained secretion of LHRH. As gestation progresses, concentrations are suppressed in the male fetus in association with the rising concentration of testosterone (Figure 9.1). However, they remain high in the female fetus. In the third phase there is suppression of gonadotrophin secretion in both male and female by the steroids of the fetoplacental unit. In the male, gonadotrophins are probably needed for the descent of the testes, particularly from the inguinal ring to the scrotum; cryptorchidism is common in patients with Kallman's syndrome, which represents a spectrum of disorders of the frequency and amplitude of hypothalamic LHRH secretion. In the female, gonadotrophins are needed for development and maturation of the ovaries, which continues throughout childhood. Anencephalic female fetuses do not have cystic ovaries. There is considerable fluctuation of gonadotrophin secretion in the first weeks of life. Thereafter concentrations remain low, although episodic secretion of low-amplitude gonadotrophin release probably continues throughout childhood. The prepubertal period is marked by sleep-related rises in gonadotrophin secretion, particularly LH, although secretion at this stage is still of low amplitude.

Figure 9.1: Changes in Hormone Levels in the Human Male *in utero*, Early Life and Thence through Childhood

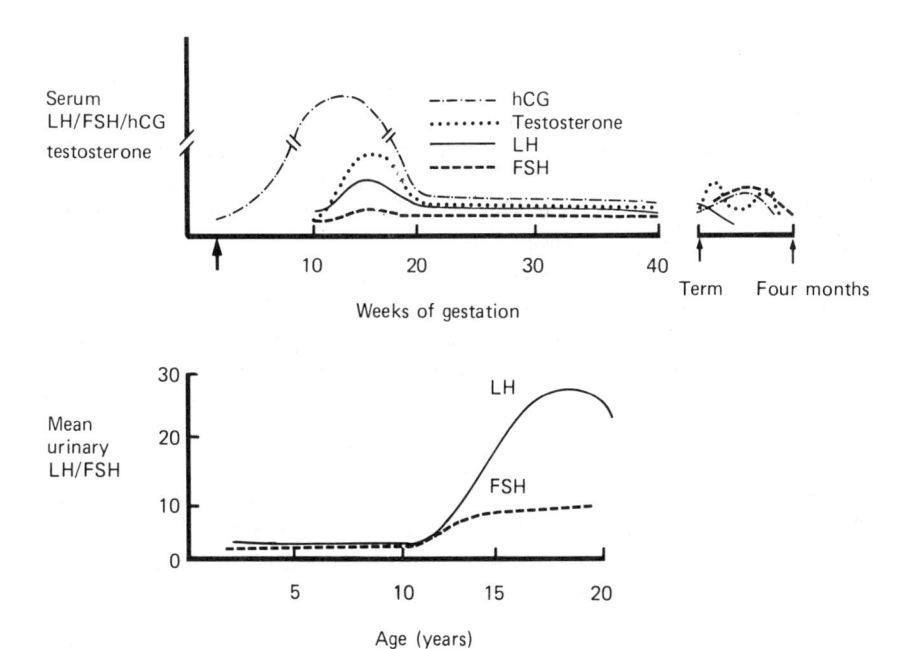

Puberty

AT the age of 8 to 10 years adrenarche occurs, with increased androgen secretion and the occasional appearance of sparse pubic hair, but there are usually no other outward manifestations except a small rise in growth velocity. Following adrenarche, gonadal maturation is accelerated. In the prepubertal period the hypothalamic output of LHRH is in some way inhibited (Figure 9.2). With the

Figure 9.2: Diagram Demonstrating the Loss of Central Inhibition of LHRH which Occurs after Puberty

PREPUBERTAL CHILD

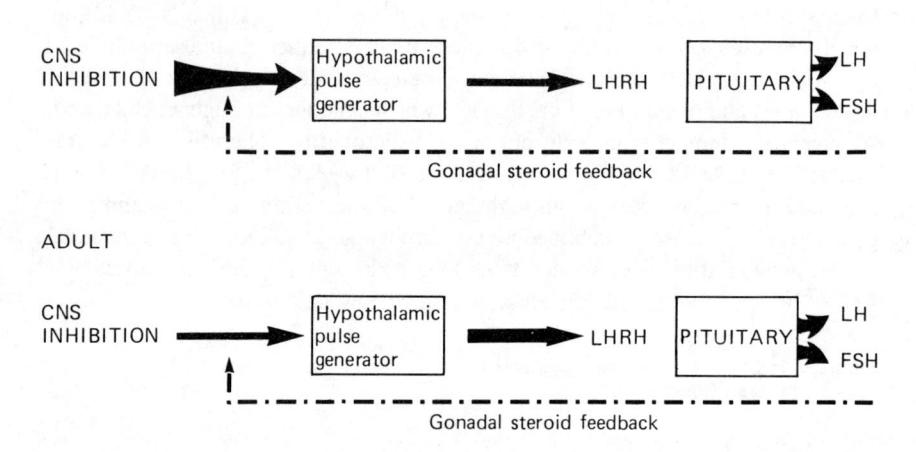

CNS INHIBITION ➡ Hypothalamic pulse generator ➡ LHRH ➡ PITUITARY ➡ LH / FSH

Gonadal steroid feedback

ADULT

CNS INHIBITION ➡ Hypothalamic pulse generator ➡ LHRH ➡ PITUITARY ➡ LH / FSH

Gonadal steroid feedback

release of this brake, pituitary gonadotrophins rise, nocturnal spikes of LH and FSH appear (and eventually occur throughout the day and night) and gonadal steroids increase. The nature of the prepubertal inhibition of LHRH release remains obscure. It was originally postulated that there was a hypothalamic 'gonadostat' that was exquisitely sensitive to steroidal feedback in childhood, but which became markedly less sensitive at the time of initiation of puberty. However, children with gonadal dysgenesis also show the prepubertal suppression of gonadotrophin levels, so interactions with gonadal steroids do not appear to be an essential part of the mechanism; in hypothalamic hypopituitarism one can mimic all the events of puberty by administering pulsatile LHRH. It is possible that pineal secretions such as melatonin and related indoles are important inhibitors of LHRH release, but the current evidence is less than convincing. Recent sophisticated analyses of gonadotrophin pulsatility have indicated that in childhood the LHRH oscillator is pulsing at normal frequency, but with a much diminished amplitude. The initiation of puberty is thus achieved by an unknown process which amplifies this invariant frequency at night. In the rat this process probably involves a stimulatory noradrenergic output, but this is almost certainly not the case in the human.

The Ovulation Cycle

The ovulation cycle is one of at least two regular reproductive cycles and refers to changes in the ovary. It is conveniently divided into two parts, the follicular phase and the luteal phase. Dependent on changes in the ovary are changes in the uterus, which relate to the menstrual cycle of 28 days' duration, which again has two phases, proliferative and secretory (Figure 9.3).

In the ovulation cycle there is a low rate of pulses of LHRH during the luteal phase, resulting in low concentrations of LH and FSH, under the impact of

The Gonadotrophins and LHRH 113

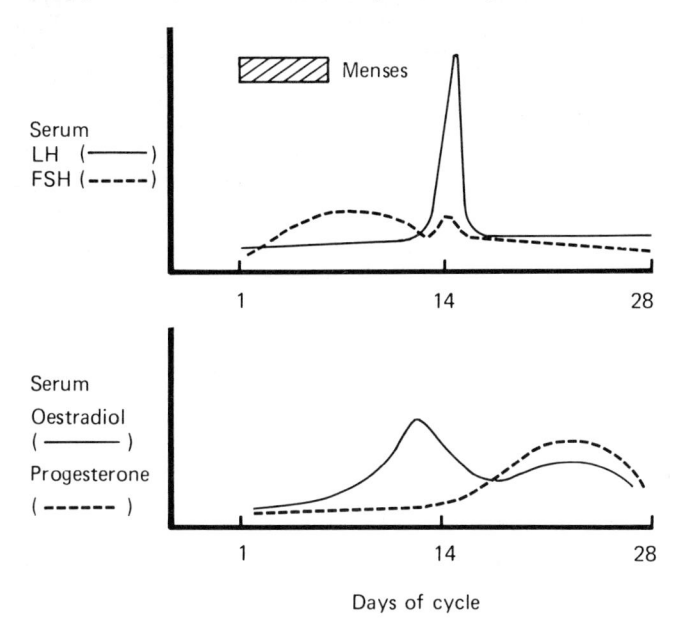

Figure 9.3: Changes in Serum LH, FSH, Oestrodiol and Progesterone during a Normal Menstrual Cycle. Ovulation occurred at day 14, shortly after the maximum LH surge

progesterone and oestrogen. With the waning of the corpus luteum there is an increase in the rate of firing of LHRH cells with a resultant increase in FSH in the early part of the follicular phase, the release being pulsatile. The gradual and incremental rise in FSH concentrations leads to follicular development and the production of inhibin. This exerts a negative feedback with decreased circulating FSH concentrations, despite the increased rate of firing of LHRH neurones. As oestradiol secretion from the developing follicle increases, the rate of LHRH pulse frequency steadily increases and oestradiol augments the response (positive feedback) so that there is a massive discharge of LH and FSH resulting in ovulation. The corpus luteum then develops with the production of progesterone (and oestradiol), which produces a low rate of LHRH firing (Figure 9.4). This allows the pituitary stores of gonadotrophins to be built up so that when the rate of pulses of LHRH increases, there is sufficient FSH present to allow for augmented release. The pattern of LH secretion is important in luteolysis. In recent data derived from patients with LHRH pumps (see below) it has been found that if the pumps are set to pulse at 90 min intervals, the luteal phase lasts its normal 14 days. If, however, the pump is withdrawn, the corpus luteum wanes. Therefore at least two factors are involved in luteolysis, the pituitary (LH) and the intrinsic genetic programme of the corpus luteum and LH receptors. It is interesting that naloxone can counteract the fall in gonadotrophin pulse frequency during the luteal phase, implying an increase in hypothalamic opioid activity at this time. The changes in LHRH pulse frequency suggests that the menstrual cycle is controlled by the hypothalamus, but in fact 28-day cycles can be maintained in patients with hypothalamic lesions and women deficient in endogenous LHRH by giving LHRH with an unvarying interval between pulses. Thus the basic 'clock' appears to depend on the complex feedback of pituitary gonadotrophin pools and gonadal steroids with a 'permissive' hypothalamic input. Nevertheless, there is a definite central variation in that the LH 'surge' invariably occurs in the early hours of the morning. In other species, particularly the rat, the neural input appears to predominate, and the oestrous cycle is under greater central control. Luteolysis in the human occurs due to a failure of human placental hCG production and the subsequent menses may in part depend on various ovarian factors such as the prostaglandins and ovarian oxytocin. Unlike in the rat, prolactin is not necessary for normal luteal function in the human. In the event of conception, placental hCG rises early and maintains the corpus luteum.

Figure 9.4: Typical Patterns of LH Pulsatility during the Midfollicular and Midluteal Phases

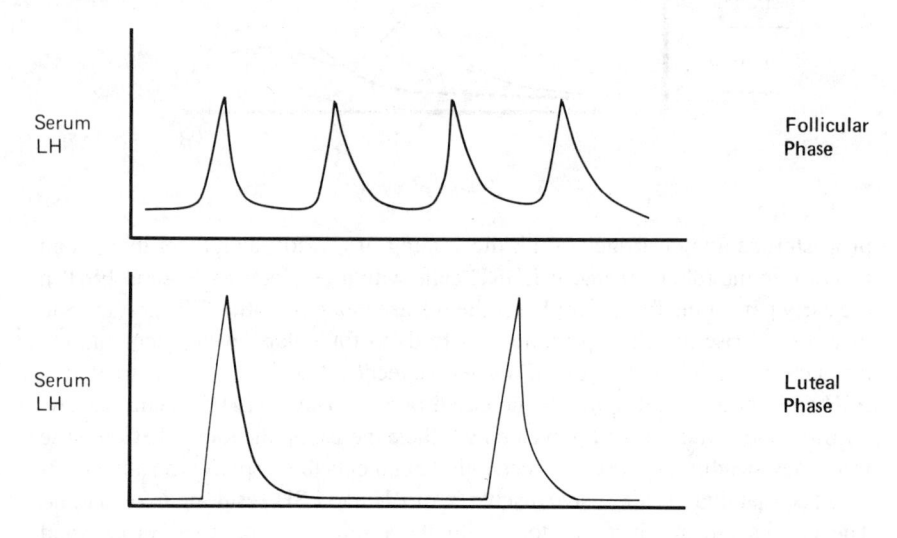

Pregnancy

Maternal LH and FSH are initially undetectable during human pregnancy, although the placental gonadotrophin (hCG) circulates, which is very similar to LH in its biological action. The oestrogens produced by the fetoplacental unit also induce lactotroph hyperplasia, so that the pituitary approximately doubles in size and serum prolactin rises in early pregnancy to 2000–4000 mU/ml. However, galactorrhoea is not noted until the puerperium, when the sudden fall in oestrogens removes the peripheral blockade to milk release. The causes and endocrine changes marking the onset of labour remain to be clarified but may possibly involve pituitary oxytocin release (see Chapter 12). The gonadotrophins remain at low levels during lactation, with cycling suppressed, at least in the post-partum period. It appears that during suckling the hypothalamic pituitary axis is more sensitive to negative feedback and relatively insensitive to positive feedback, possibly secondary to the hyperprolactinaemia at this time. Ovulation rarely occurs as long as suckling continues and no supplemenetary foods are introduced. Once non-maternal feeding is initiated, the stimulus to prolactin secretion decreases and irregular cycling supervenes. It is important to realise that the first cycle may indeed be ovulatory and a further pregnancy may ensue without an intervening menstrual flow.

The Menopause

By the end of reproductive life almost all of the ovarian follicles have disappeared with a decline in ovarian activity. The ovarian secretion of the major ovarian hormones finally stops at the menopause at about 50 years of age. The negative feedback of the ovarian hormones disappears almost completely, with a resultant greatly increased secretion of LH and FSH. The highest levels are seen in the age group 51–60 years, the FSH levels being about 10 times higher than during the reproductive age and the mean LH concentration four times higher. In comparison with the midcycle peak, the LH concentrations after menopause are about a third as high and those for FSH are 10 times greater. This is followed by a gradual decline in serum LH and FSH levels in later life.

Release in the Male

Gonadotrophins in the male are also released in a pulsatile fashion: the characteristic pattern seems to be a rapid secretion over a 10 to 15-minute period followed by a decrease, the cycle occurring every two hours. The FSH pulses are much lower in amplitude than those of LH. There is evidence that gonadotrophin concentrations increase with age, probably as a result of altered testicular function. Studies on infusions of various sex steroids in man have demonstrated that testosterone probably feeds back on to the hypothalamo-pituitary axis via conversion to active metabolites. It seems likely that aromatisation to oestrogen is effective in suppressing pulse amplitude and this could occur (at least in part) at the level of the pituitary. On the other hand, reduction to dihydrotestosterone causes changes in the pulse frequency, presumably at a suprapituitary level. Thus the mean levels of serum LH and FSH seen in normal men are dependent on the effects of metabolic conversion of testosterone by at least two processes at two sites with the resultant frequency and amplitude modulated pulses. Under such circumstances it is surprising that single random levels are so clinically useful.

Action of the Gonadotrophins

(A) In the Female

LH acts on the cells of the ovarian stroma and theca to cause an increase in steroidogenesis by stimulating the conversion of cholesterol, the precursor molecule of all steroids, to pregnenolone, an intermediate in the synthesis of progesterone. The initial step is an interaction of LH with the membrane receptors on the responsive cells. This is followed by activation of adenylate cyclase, resulting in an increase in intracellular cyclic AMP. The effect of LH is probably mediated, at least in part, by the interaction of cyclic AMP with cellular processes such as activation of protein phosphorylation mechanisms. The principal steroid produced by the ovarian theca is testosterone, which is transferred to the granulosa cells in the follicle where it is aromatised to oestradiol under the influence of FSH. Just before ovulation, there is an increase of LH receptors in the granulosa cells of the follicle, which in turn become steroidogenic and secrete progesterone. Following ovulation, the corpus luteum containing granulosa and trapped theca cells remains steroidogenic and produces both oestradiol and progesterone. Thus the function of the corpus luteum is maintained by LH. Binding of LH has also been noted in corpora lutea in the first trimester and in term pregnancies, but at a lower level than during the cycle.

FSH stimulates follicular development in the ovary and this effect is augmented by oestrogen and LH. Serum FSH is high during menstruation (i.e. the first part of the follicular phase) and then progressively declines until mid-cycle. This fall may be attributed to the rising oestrogen concentration and/or an increase in inhibin. The granulosa cells are the primary site of follicular oestrogen production and FSH regulates oestrogen secretion by acting on the aromatisation of androgen. Under the influence of the early rise of FSH, the primary follicles develop into secondary follicles. Normally, only one of the follicles develops into a mature follicle, the remainder undergoing regression (or atresia) possibly due to the falling FSH levels. It appears that the 'window' at which FSH is rising will usually only find one follicle in the correct stage of development. The selected follicle develops a progressively larger oocyte and the surrounding granulosa cells proliferate and secrete progressively larger amounts of oestradiol to reach a peak just prior to the LH/FSH surge. Progesterone levels rise in parallel with the LH ovulatory surge. At ovulation the follicle ruptures and releases the ovum. The empty follicle becomes a corpus luteum in which the thecal cells are entrapped between granulosa cells. The corpus luteum continues to produce oestrogen and progesterone under the influence of LH for 10 to 16 days following ovulation and then undergoes regression (luteolysis), possibly because the LH level reaches a minimum in response to the negative feedback exerted by oestrogen.

(B) In the Male

The secretion of the two major testicular steroid hormones and the process of spermatogenesis are segregated anatomically, androgen biosynthesis occurring in the Leydig cells and spermatogenesis in the seminiferous tubules. Both LH and FSH are required for spermatogenesis, the former exerting its effects via testosterone. LH acts to stimulate testosterone secretion; its mode of action is analogous to that in the ovary (see above). FSH acts synergistically with LH in this regard in some species. During sexual maturation FSH causes an increase in the LH receptors on Leydig cells and induces responsiveness to LH. In the adult, LH appears to be the major modulator of testosterone secretion. FSH is necessary for spermatogenesis, but it is only a transitory effect limited to the development of the spermatids. Thereafter spermatogenesis is maintained by androgen secreted from the Leydig cells in response to LH. The sites of FSH action are the Sertoli cells, which are stimulated to produce an androgen binding protein. The action of FSH appears to be mediated by adenylate cyclase. The androgen binding protein interacts with androgen which has diffused from the interstitial area, thereby resulting in a high androgen concentration in the vicinity of the germ cells (androgen binding protein can be induced and maintained by testosterone). The Sertoli cells are thought to secrete a peptide known as inhibin, which feeds back to inhibit pituitary FSH release; the presence of such a substance was originally suggested to explain the observation that the rise in FSH induced by gonadectomy is not totally blocked by physiological levels of oestrogens or progesterone.

Assays

The gonadotrophins may be assayed in several systems. One general problem is that since both LH and FSH are secreted in pulses, a single sample may not be representative of the basal level. Conventional bioassays such as the augmentation of hCG-stimulated ovarian weight and testosterone production by mouse Leydig cells (for LH) have now been largely superseded by radioimmunoassays and radioreceptor assays. Relatively specific radioimmunoassays have been developed for both gonadotrophins, although most antisera against LH also react with hCG. In the more recently developed radioreceptor assays LH may be assayed using Leydig cell membranes, ovarian homogenates and plasma membranes as binding reagents, and FSH may be measured using the specific hormone receptors on rat seminiferous tubule membranes.

Clinical Disorders

Overproduction of Gonadotrophins

Primary hypogonadism is often accompanied by increased plasma gonadotrophin concentrations as a result of the lack of feedback inhibition in both female and male subjects. Patients with Turner's syndrome (XO karyotype) may have high gonadotrophin levels in the first four years of life and certainly after 10 years of age. Raised serum concentrations of LH and suppressed FSH are well recognised in the polycystic ovary syndrome. The amplitude and the frequency of LH pulses are increased, and it has been suggested that this may be related to the positive feedback of certain oestrogens, particularly oestrone. Increased gonadotrophin secretion may also accompany hypersecreting adenomas of the pituitary but such 'gonadotrophinomas' are very rare.

Generally speaking, elevated levels of both gonadotrophins in a single sample imply loss of gonadal feedback and therefore gonadal failure. Very occasionally, high gonadotrophin levels are seen in women with relatively normal levels of plasma oestradiol and such patients may have the 'resistant ovary syndrome'.

Excess oestrogen therapy may paradoxically reduce ovarian 'resistance'. However, even high gonadotrophin levels do not necessarily imply the termination of all gonadal activity, as waxing and waning of ovarian function can be seen in the perimenopausal period, and conception has been achieved at this time. A very elevated serum LH with a relatively normal serum FSH usually denotes either polycystic ovary syndrome, or that the patient was sampled during ovulation. Single serum samples for gonadotrophins must always be interpreted in the light of the phase of the menstrual cycle, the pulsatile nature of their secretion and the prevailing steroid milieu. Thus low-normal levels of LH and FSH in a young thin woman with low-normal plasma oestradiol suggests a weight-related hypothalamic defect; elevated gonadotrophin levels in a young man with low or borderline testosterone indicates primary gonadal failure, and Klinefelter's syndrome also needs to be considered.

Underproduction of Gonadotrophins

Isolated gonadotrophin deficiency has often been described, and is normally associated with the lack of both LH and FSH although there are reports of isolated LH and FSH deficiencies. In women with bihormonal deficiency there are symptoms of amenorrhoea and some atrophy of the secondary sexual characteristics. In the male there is failure to develop secondary sexual characteristics and infertility. A lack of LH alone has been described in males only and results in poorly developed secondary sexual characteristics, although development of the seminiferous tubules and spermatogenesis is normal. Isolated FSH deficiency has been reported to lead to amenorrhoea and lack of follicle development in the female, and to germinal cell aplasia in the male. If the hypogonadotrophic deficiencies are hypothalamic in origin, treatment with LHRH may be successful (see below). Failure of gonadotrophin secretion may be congenital as in Kallman's syndrome in which there are disorders in the rate of firing of LHRH cells variably associated with deafness, colour blindness and defects of olfaction. The other priniciple condition in which there may be low serum gonadotrophin concentrations is anorexia nervosa, in which the low weight is associated with a return to a prepubertal gonadal status.

The Use of LHRH in Diagnostic Testing

Administration of native or synthetic LHRH (a decapeptide) to animals or human subjects can result in a rapid increase in serum LH and FSH, reaching a peak level at around 30 min and then declining to normal values after 1–2 h. Like TRH, LHRH has a relatively short half-life in the circulation. In general, however, the response to exogenous LHRH depends not only on the dose, method and route of administration of the hormone, but also on the background of steroid hormones. Whereas infusion is equally effective in releasing LH and FSH, a single bolus injection is more effective in releasing LH. The releasing hormone also appears to have a self-priming action at the level of the pituitary in that a second dose is more effective than the first. This is dependent on the timing of the doses as the pituitary is desensitised after prolonged exposure or after repeated LHRH injections. These responses appear to depend on the presence of a readily releasable pool, which can be equated with pituitary sensitivity, and a non-releasable pool, which can be equated with pituitary reserve and which requires sustained LHRH stimulation. In rhesus monkeys, pulsatile infusion of releasing hormone releases FSH and LH whereas a continuous infusion leads to a loss of response. In the human there is considerable variation in the response to LHRH during the menstrual cycle, with increased responsiveness during the late follicular phase and around the time of ovulation.

The acute response to a single bolus of LHRH is a widely used test of pituitary gonadotrophin function, but essentially only assesses the readily releasable pool. A normal response with a marked rise in serum LH and a smaller rise in FSH is useful as a rapid test of pituitary function. However, a poor response may either indicate that there is defective gonadotroph function or that the pituitary has not been recently primed with LHRH, implying that there is a hypothalamic defect. Occasionally, successive doses of exogenous LHRH may be given to prime the pituitary and demonstrate a normal pituitary reserve. Similarly, priming, using prolonged pulsatile delivery of LHRH, may also normalise the defective acute responses to LHRH often seen in patients with weight-related menstrual disorders such as anorexia nervosa.

Excessive gonadotrophin responses to LHRH may be seen when the basal levels are elevated, and also in many patients with hyperprolactinaemia. Such patients inhibit the regular pulsatile secretion of LHRH, but probably enough is transferred via the portal vessels such that the pituitary reserve is equal to or greater than normal.

In general, the LHRH test is most useful in excluding gross pituitary pathology in women with amenorrhoea. In such patients further testing with clomiphene may reveal a hypothalamic defect. Clomiphene, a synthetic anti-oestrogen, is thought to stimulate hypothalamic LHRH release in normal subjects as LH either doubles or rises outside the normal range in the standard test. It may also have an action at the pituitary level (see Chapter 14). Thus a normal response to LHRH but no response to clomiphene implies that there is a functional hypothalamic defect, and is characteristic of Kallman's syndrome and weight-related amenorrhoea. In prepubertal children and more severe cases of anorexia nervosa, there may be a blunted response to LHRH, often with a greater FSH than LH response and a *fall* in the gonadotrophins after clomiphene. The latter phenomenon is thought to be due to the drug's intrinsic oestrogen agonist activity.

There is no diagnostic value in the timing of the peak gonadotrophin response to LHRH.

LHRH as a Therapeutic Agent

Early studies showed that repeated injections of LHRH could establish normal sex function and fertility in men with Kallman's syndrome and could restore menstrual regularity in women with anorexia nervosa. However, repeated subcutaneous injections are obviously inconvenient, so the introduction of superactive analogues of LHRH (with amino acid substitutions to increase resistance to enzymic degradation) was heralded as a new era in the treatment of fertility. It was, however, rapidly discovered that such analogues rapidly *decreased* gonadal function following a short-lived stimulation. Indeed, such analogues, probably because of their persistent receptor occupancy, downregulate the pituitary receptors and block cyclic gonadotrophin release. There are, however, several promising potential therapeutic uses for such agents. In men with carcinoma of the prostate, the androgen dependency of the tumour has led to the frequent use of stilboestrol therapy. Unfortunately, the decreased mortality from the primary cancer has been matched by an increased mortality from oestrogen-related cardiovascular complications. Analogues of LHRH given either by intranasal spray or daily (or even monthly) depot injection decrease gonadal function within a week or two and have led to remarkable disease remissions. Nevertheless, further work is required to assess the relative importance of adrenal androgen production.

LHRH analogues are also highly effective in the treatment of hypothalamic isosexual precocious puberty, a rare disorder in which puberty occurs early in childhood, often before 5 years of age (see below). Other potential uses for LHRH analogues include the prevention of ovulation in normal women — a non-steroidal contraceptive — and the abolition of menstrual cycles where it is desirable to minimise gonadal activity as in endometriosis, oestrogen-dependent neoplasms and acute porphyria variegata. In all these conditions LHRH is thought to act solely by downregulation of the pituitary, unlike the situation in the rat where LHRH may have an extrapituitary effect, acting directly on the gonads.

In patients deficient in LHRH where an increase in pulsatile gonadotrophic activity is desired, the conventional treatment has been either with clomiphene (when there is a functional defect in LHRH release) or with gonadotrophin therapy. The structure of clomiphene citrate, first introduced in 1960, bears some similarity to diethylstilboestrol and it is thought that it may act competitively by inhibiting the action of oestrogen at the hypothalmic or pituitary level. Of course, for the treatment to be successful, the pituitary needs to be capable of secreting gonadotrophins. These have been used since 1930 when Cole and Hunt isolated pregnant-mare serum gonadotrophins. Gemzell and his colleagues first reported the use of human pituitary FSH, but supplies were limited until the commercial development of the production of gonadotrophin from the urine of post-menopausal women ('Pergonal'). Treatment with human menopausal gonadotrophin is followed by administration of human chorionic gonadotrophin, used to replace the normal LH surge. The dose of human menopausal gonadotrophin required to produce a satisfactory response varies from individual to individual so that the response must be monitored by determining the secretion of oestrogen. Conventional Pergonal contains equal amounts of FSH and LH, but the recent development of relatively pure human FSH may change treatment strategies.

Unfortunately, gonadotrophin therapy is extremely expensive, requires close patient co-operation over many months, and even in centres of excellence is reported as having a hyperstimulation rate of 3 per cent and a multiple conception

The Gonadotrophins and LHRH 121

Figure 9.5: Mean Serum Concentrations of LH and FSH and the Follicular Diameter during the Ovulation Induced in Women with Hypothalamic Amenorrhoea by Pulsatile Administration of LHRH. (Taken from Mason *et al.* (1982), *British Medical Journal*, *288*, 181-5; reproduced with permission of the authors and the Editor of the *British Medical Journal*.)

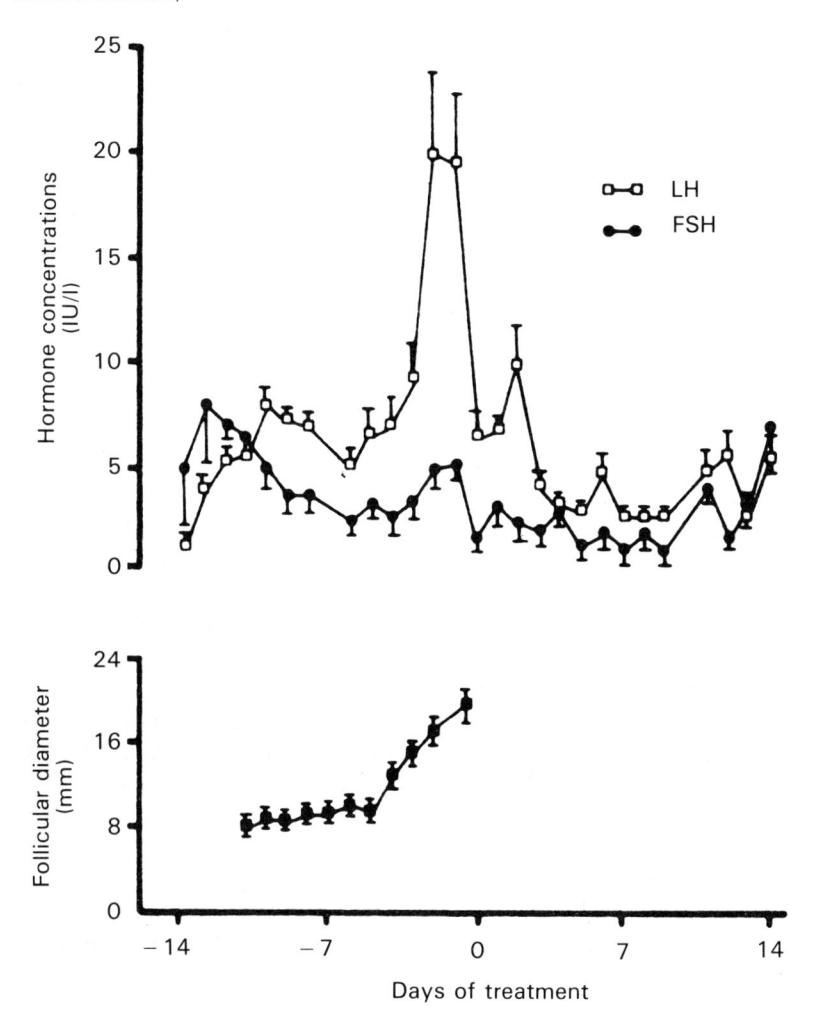

rate of 20 per cent (this figure may, however, be considerably lowered by extra-careful supervision). Synthetic native LHRH may be given by means of a miniature infusion pump and there are now several clinical trials of its use in treating men and women with functional defects in LHRH release. Intravenous administration has its hazards, but in some trials administration of 90-minute subcutaneous boluses of 5–15 µg native LHRH has been highly successful in the induction of menstruation and eventual fertility (Figure 9.5). Of course, the nature of treatment precludes its long-term use, but for the short-term use in promoting fertility with ultrasound monitoring it may become the treatment of choice in Kallman's syndrome. Patients with functional defects in LHRH release frequently have weight-related menstrual disorders, and it is possible that sufficient weight gain would obviate the need for such treatment. Equally, patients with the polycystic ovary syndrome are generally unresponsive to pulsatile LHRH therapy. Nevertheless, LHRH pumps will undoubtedly play an important role in the therapy of infertility in the future.

Delayed and Precocious Puberty

Puberty is a process that occurs over a period of years: the age at which it occurs varies with individuals. However, the onset of pubertal signs below the age of 8 years in girls or 9 years in boys definitely merits investigation, as does their complete absence at 13.8 years in girls and 14.0 years in boys. Pubertal development is graded via a series of stages occurring in a certain sequence to give normal consonance to puberty. As already indicated, the onset of puberty is normally heralded by adrenarche. In boys this is subsequently followed by an increase in testicular growth, the first sign of puberty in a boy, and penile growth, increased muscle development, body hair and deepening of the voice. In girls the first sign of puberty is breast development (thelarche). Then follows redistribution of body fat and ultimately the appearance of the first menstrual period (menarche). However, it should be realised that this is not the end of the process, as non-ovulatory cycles usually predominate well into the next two years.

In isosexual precocious puberty, any of these stages may occur independently with loss of consonance of normal puberty, i.e. pseudopuberty. However, the most frequent finding is for the whole pubertal process to be prematurely activated, i.e. true or central precocious puberty. In girls, the great majority of such cases are 'idiopathic', and no obvious structural abnormality can be established even with high-resolution CT scanning. The premature onset of puberty is often associated with emotional and social problems; the premature closure of the bone epiphyses severely limits adult height. Endocrine function is generally in accord with the pubertal stage, with the appearance of nocturnal then night-and-day LH pulses, an increase in the LH response to LHRH, and a progressive rise in plasma oestradiol. It is important to differentiate isosexual precocious puberty from feminising tumours, usually of ovarian or adrenal origin: abdominal CT scan or pelvic ultrasound should localise the lesion. Some female patients with congenital adrenal hyperplasia may also present during childhood, but the early adrenarche (pseudopuberty) will then progress to further virilisation.

In boys, isosexual precocious puberty is more commonly associated with intracranial disease, especially with raised intracranial pressure, and a suprasellar tumour such as a germinoma must always be excluded. These rare tumours (see Chapter 4) arise from germinal elements in the pineal or anterior hypothalamus, and may accelerate puberty by disrupting the normal inhibition of LHRH release or, by the ectopic secretion of hCG. The tumours are usually readily visible on a CT scan and are frequently associated with field defects and abnormalities in eye movement, particularly Peyrinaud's triad (failure of upgaze, convergent nystagmus and Argyll-Robertson pupils). It is probable that some of the so-called 'idiopathic' cases of precocious puberty in boys are also associated with structural defects, such as hypothalamic hamartomas. Virilising tumours require exclusion, especially when testicular development is less marked than other indices of puberty. Optic gliomas or any other tumour in this area can also be associated with precocious puberty, as can (rarely) radiotherapy.

In the McCune-Albright syndrome, isosexual precocious puberty is associated with polyostotic fibrous dysplasia and abnormal areas of skin pigmentation. At least part of the precocious puberty is due to premature activation of the pituitary-gonadal axis, although there may be abnormal development of the gonad itself. The very rare 'testotoxicosis' presents as isosexual precocious puberty in boys, and is independent of hypothalamo-pituitary activation: the aetiology remains completely unknown.

The treatment of precocious puberty remains a problem in both boys and girls. The mainstay of treatment in the past has been cyproterone acetate, which works, at least in part, by blocking the hypothalamo-gonadal axis. It also interferes with gonadal steroid synthesis, and is an androgen-receptor antagonist. Large doses may need to be given, and are rarely completely effective. The acceleration in bone maturation is particularly difficult to control. In addition, cyproterone acetate has corticosteroid-like activity and may cause suppression of the pituitary-adrenal axis, thus necessitating treating such children with hydrocortisone cover during surgical procedures and severe infections. Recently, the analogues of LHRH have been used to cause inhibition of pituitary gonadotrophin release. As with other disease states such as prostatic cancer, these analogues may be administered by nasal spray several times daily, by daily subcutaneous injection, or possibly by 4 to 6 weekly depot injections. Provisional data are encouraging, although combination therapy with cyproterone acetate may be necessary during the early weeks of treatment to avoid the consequences of the transient initial stimulation of gonadotrophin release. It is currently uncertain, however, as to the degree of reversibility of the induced gonadal regression, and until the results of long-term trials are available, the shortest duration of therapy should be aimed at. Follow-up of children treated with cyproterone acetate has demonstrated normal development and fertility subsequently, with attained height not too restricted, especially in children going into puberty over the age of 5 years.

Delayed puberty is a more common problem, and is usually part of a generalised delay in the developmental process. Constitutional delay is a problem in boys because the growth spurt occurs only towards the end of puberty at the attainment of a 10 ml testicular volume. Often there will be a family history of delayed puberty and a retarded bone age; the latter will usually allow the prediction of a good adult height. Detailed tables are available for the calculation of bone age and predicted height, although some skill is required in their detailed administration. Computerisation is undoubtedly helpful in this context, and has even been applied to direct interpretation of radiographs. Wrist and lower forearm radiographs are standard, with supplementation of iliac crest and sternal clavicle views in older children and adolescents. Children with constitutional delayed puberty are often thin, quite unlike the 'chubby' appearance of true GH-deficient children. In cases of doubt, GH stimulated tests may be appropriate, usually using either insulin or clonidine.

Occasionally, marginally subnormal GH repesonses to provocative stimuli occur in the peripubertal period, and may be normalised by 'priming' with gonadal steroids (usually stilboestrol) for several days. As GH responses to GHRH are not altered by priming, it appears that the steroids are probably acting at a hypothalamic level.

Almost any form of non-endocrine disease may present as delayed puberty, and such patients may also present as failure to thrive. Most of these cases will be obvious, although various forms of gastrointestinal disease in particular may be quite occult. Any form of abdominal pain should alert one to the possibility of Crohn's disease, and a sedimentation rate should form part of a standard screen for all such children. A suspicion of gluten-sensitive enteropathy requires assessment of the serum folate, and a jejunal biopsy should be considered at an early stage.

The chromosomal disorders of Klinefelter's syndrome (XXY) and Turner's syndrome (XO) may present as delayed puberty, but do not usually cause problems in diagnosis. In Klinefelter's syndrome there is excessive growth, a eunuchoid habitus and very small firm testes; girls with Turner's syndrome will usually have the other somatic manifestations of this condition. In both instances, elevated circulating levels of the gonadotrophins are invariably present at this stage. It should be noted that some girls may lack many of the other features of Turner's syndrome if they are XX/XO mosaics, and careful karyotyping in a specialist centre is mandatory in girls with primary gonadal dysgenesis. Noonan's syndrome usually refers to the somatic manifestations of Turner's syndrome in the presence of a normal chromosomal complement, plus or minus gonadal dysgenesis, and may occur in males. Other congenital abnormalities involving hypogonadism include the Lawrence-Moon-Biedl syndrome (obesity, polydactyly hypogonadism, mental retardation, retinitis pigmentosa), the Prader-Willi syndrome (gross obesity, hypogonadism, plus other dysmorphic features) and dystrophia myotonica: all are very rare. Space-occupying lesions of the pituitary and hypothalamus are also rare causes of delayed puberty, and usually act by decreasing gonadotrophin release, although a raised serum prolactin may also cause arrest of pubertal progression. Increasingly, anorexia nervosa may present as delayed puberty or primary amenorrhoea in young girls, and should always be considered even in the presence of a 'normal' dietary history.

Normal puberty takes 2 to 3 years, and in 3 per cent of children up to 5 years, so that in treatment one should ideally try to mimic this time scale. In males, human hCG may be given in small amounts, e.g. 500 U intramuscularly twice a week, and then increased gradually. This will usually produced a testicular size that plateaus at 7-8 ml (normal $c.$ 20 ml), and may then be replaced by testosterone therapy, initially also at a low dose. Although hCG increases intratesticular testosterone production and thus aids spermatogenesis, full testicular growth and a normal seminal fluid analysis requires some form of FSH. On grounds of cost for the currently available forms, this can only be recommended for induction of fertility when required. Replacement therapy in girls should also be introduced in small amounts, with oestrogen given in a daily dose around 5 μg initially. Cyclical oestrogen therapy may be introduced after a year, and finally adult replacement therapy (ethinyloestradiol 20–30 μg daily for 3 weeks, medroxyprogesterone acetate 5 mg daily for one week) may be introduced. Pulsatile subcutaneous LHRH therapy is certainly effective and is a more 'physiological' way to initiate puberty, but is unlikely ever to be convenient and acceptable enough to the majority of patients. In cases of constitutional delay, reassurance alone is sufficient for most children and their parents. However, where social or psychological function is becoming disordered, 1 or 2 years of therapy may be useful to initiate the process. Kallman's syndrome, or 'idiopathic isolated LHRH deficiency', may often only be differentiated from constitutional pubertal delay by a trial of therapy followed by observation of the patient in the absence of treatment.

Further Reading

Belchetz, P.E. (1983) 'Gonadotrophin Regulation and Clinical Applications of GnRH', *Clinics in Endocrinology and Metabolism, 12*, 619–40

Butt, W.R. (1983) 'Gonadotrophins', in C.H. Gray and V.H.T James (eds), *Hormones in Blood*, 3rd edition, Vol. 4, pp. 148–77, Academic Press, New York

Filicori, M. and Crowley, W.F. (1984) 'Hypothalamic Regulation of Gonadotrophin Secretion in Women', in R.L. Norman (ed.), *Neuroendocrine Aspects of Reproduction*, pp. 185–294, Academic Press, New York

Franks, S. (1981) 'Male Reproductive Endocrinology', *Clinics in Obstetrics and Gynaecology, 8*, 549–70

McCann, S.M. (1983) 'Progress in Neuroendocrinology; LH Releasing Factor (LHRH), Basic and Clinical Aspects', *Journal of Endocrinological Investigation, 6*, 243–51

Reiter, O.E. and Grumbach, M.M. (1982) 'Neuroendocrine Mechanisms and the Onset of Puberty', *Annual Review of Physiology, 44*, 595–613

Waxman, J. (1985) 'Hormonal Aspects of Prostatic Cancer: a Review', *Journal of the Royal Society of Medicine, 78*, 129–35

Yen, S.S.C. (1983) 'Clinical Applications of Gonadotrophin Releasing Hormone and Gonadotrophin Releasing Hormone Analogs', *Fertility and Sterility, 39*, 257–66

10 THYROTROPHIN RELEASING HORMONE AND THYROID STIMULATING HORMONE

Historical Background

Parry, Graves and von Basedow independently recognised a syndrome now termed Graves' disease, features of which were tachycardia, intense nervousness, tremor, enlargement of the thyroid and exophthalmos. In 1886 Mobius suggested that a pathological alteration in the thyroid gland was the basis of the condition. In 1874 Gull connected the symptoms of myxoedema with atrophy of the thyroid, and this, together with other observations, established the thyroid as a gland involved in the control of many body functions. That control of the thyroid was via the pituitary took some time to establish. In 1851, Niepe had noted an enlargement of the pituitary in association with parenchymous goitre in animals and man. Later, Regowitsch showed in rabbits that thyroidectomy resulted in obvious enlargement of the pituitary. At the beginning of the present century, Adler, in heroic studies in which he attempted the hypophysectomy of 12 000 tadpoles, showed that removal of the pituitary gland resulted in atrophy of the thyroid gland and failure of metamorphosis. Some twenty years later Smith showed that extracts of bovine pituitary glands would stimulate thyroid secretion in hypophysectomised tadpoles and later confirmed the observation in rats. It was not until the 1930s and 1940s that bioassays were developed for the pituitary thyroid stimulating hormone. Many approaches were used, based on the various aspects of thyroid function.

It must, however, be stated that in the early 1930s there was no general agreement that there was a separate hormone which stimulated the thyroid. Riddle and his co-workers believed that the thyroid stimulating activity was produced by gonadotrophin stimulating hormones, whereas Evans and his collaborators maintained that growth hormone was responsible. As with other glycoprotein hormones, extraction and purification presented considerable problems, and for many years preparations were contaminated with other proteins including LH. An important step forward was made in 1956 when Condliffe and Bates introduced cation and anion chromatography. The final purification of thyroid stimulating hormone (TSH) was achieved in 1969 by Liao and collaborators, and the structure was eventually determined by Pearce *et al.* in 1971.

Structure of TSH

Although the specific structure of TSH varies in different species, in all it is a glycoprotein hormone and, like LH and FSH, consists of two associated polypeptide subunits, α and β. As already discussed, the α-subunit is common to the other two glycoprotein hormones, and the β-subunit confers the specific biological properties of the hormone. Human pituitary TSH has a molecular weight of 28 000 and appears to be identical to the principal circulating form, which has a half-life of 60 min. However, TSH circulates with a heterogeneity of size and structure. Free α and β-subunits are also secreted in small amounts; secretion of the β-subunit closely follows secretion of intact TSH.

Measurement of TSH

A number of bioassays have been developed, including *in vivo* tests based on thyroid weight in guinea pigs, and uptake of isotopically-labelled phosphorus or iodine by the thyroid of a number of animal preparations, including guinea pigs or hypophysectomised rats. *In vitro* assays have depended *inter alia* on blocking of a normally-occurring loss of weight by bovine thyroid tissue slices during overnight incubation, ^{32}P uptake by bovine thyroid slices and a variety of *in vivo* ^{131}I depletion uptake assays in thyroid tissue slices. Radioimmunoassays have been developed which are sensitive enough to detect basal plasma concentrations of approximately 50 pg/ml. The specificity of the individual assay depends on the use of an antiserum raised against either the α- or β-subunit.

Release of TSH

The rate of TSH secretion is determined by the stimulating effect of thyroid releasing hormone (TRH) and the inhibitory effect of circulating thyroid hormones. These opposing hormones appear to control release by competing at the pituitary thyrotroph. As with other pituitary hormones, secretion is episodic, peaks occurring every 2–4 h with maximum secretion at around 22.00 and lowest values at 11.00. The major external stimuli are changes in ambient temperature, stress and the day-night cycle. Decreased ambient temperature stimulates release, whereas increased ambient temperature and stress inhibit it. Although TSH release is markedly elevated on acute exposure to cold, changes occurrring within 10 min, and although the importance of the pituitary-thyroid axis in response to *prolonged* exposure to cold is now well documented, the absolute changes are relatively slight. The response is abolished by lesions of the hypothalamus, and temperature-mediated changes are thought to occur via changes in TRH. Extra-hypothalamic regions have also been implicated in both this and the stress response. Such regions include the habenular, pineal, extra pyramidal and limbic structures. The response to stress depends on the nature of the stimulus and, in addition to the hypothalamo-pituitary axis, may involve changes in the carrier binding proteins and peripheral metabolism of thyroid hormones. For example, it appears that during stress thyroxine conversion to tri-iodothyronine is inhibited and more of the inactive form of tri-iodothyronine (T_3), reverse T_3, is synthesised. Certain drugs have a similar effect (Figure 10.1).

Figure 10.1: The Effect of Drugs that Block the Conversion of T_4 to T_3. These changes may be useful clinically in the case of propranolol and propylthiouracil, but may raise problems in patients on the cardiac anti-arrhythmic, amiodarone

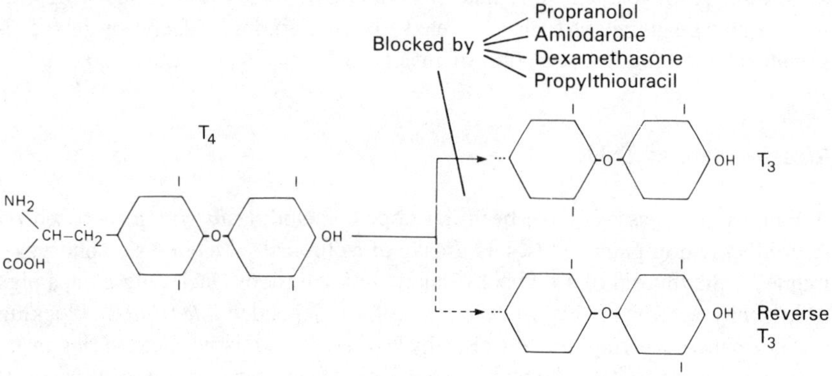

In common with other trophic hormones, secretions of the target organs (the thyroid) feed back to control the release of TSH forming a self-regulatory neuro-endocrine system. The system appears very sensitive as only very small changes in plasma thyroxine (T_4 or T_3) are needed to influence TSH secretion. Thus serum concentrations of TSH may remain remarkably constant for prolonged periods of time. This stable regulatory system can be overridden by TRH. For example, as already indicated, exposure to cold results in a sudden outpouring of TSH, an effect which can be mimicked by intravenous infusion of TRH. However, these responses can be blocked by elevating the circulating concentrations of thyroid hormones. Such results suggest competition at the level of the thyrotroph between TSH and thyroid hormones. Thus at least one site for negative feedback of thyroid hormones appears to be the pituitary gland. Although most data suggest that the principal form of feedback is by T_3 binding to nuclear receptors, it is possible that this may also occur via intrapituitary conversion of T_4 to T_3. Thus both circulating T_5 and T_3 are important mediators of feedback regulation. There is evidence from reduced TSH secretion following implantation of T_4 in the hypothalamus to suggest that T_4 also feeds back at this level, almost certainly via conversion to T_3. Two other hypothalamic factors, dopamine and somatostatin, exert inhibitory influences on TSH secretion at the level of the pituitary thyrotroph in man, which may also be of physiological importance. Whereas there is little available information on the role of somatostatin, in recent years there has been extensive study of the dopaminergic control of TSH release. The use of dopamine antagonists has revealed a marked circadian rhythm of inhibition of TSH by dopamine, with greatest inhibition at the time of the highest TSH levels, i.e. around midnight. This inhibition is more pronounced in patients with mild primary hypothyroidism. Most importantly, there is a significant increase in dopaminergic tone in patients with prolactinomas, suggesting that tumour-induced hyperprolactinaemia increases hypothalamic dopamine inhibition of the surrounding normal pituitary. Although it has been proposed that this increased tone is absent in patients with so-called functional hyperprolactinaemia, careful analysis reveals a graded increase in dopaminergic inhibition of TSH release as the level of prolactin rises. The increase in dopamine inhibition of TSH release in patients with prolactinomas may lead to a rise in thyrotroph TSH content, and may possibly account for the enhanced TSH response to TRH often seen in these patients. TSH secretion and responsiveness to TRH may also be modulated by circulating sex steroids and growth hormone.

Since thyroid hormones exert negative feedback primarily at the level of the pituitary gland, and other factors also have an inhibitory effect at this site, it seems that the hypothalamus exerts a primary stimulatory effect. The nature of hypothalamic control has been clearly demonstrated. Whereas surgical interruption of the connections between the hypothalamus and pituitary results in reduced thyroid hormone production, preparation of hypothalamic islands (in which connections of the hypothalamus to and from the rest of the brain are severed while pituitary connections remain intact) results in relatively normal TSH levels. When it became possible to stain cell bodies in the rat hypothalamus for TRH, it was found that destruction of these resulted in a 70 per cent depletion of hypothalamic TRH and consequent hypothyroidism. Secretion of TSH following TRH infusion can be mimicked by electrical stimulation of electrodes implanted in the preoptic area, or in the paraventricular, dorsomedial or ventromedial nuclei. More recently, in a study employing small surgical rather than electrical lesions, evidence was obtained that the paraventricular and periventricular nuclei are of particular importance in sustaining TSH secretion, and the medial preoptic area acts tonically to inhibit TSH release. Since this latter is an area rich in somatostatin-containing neurones, it has been postulated that the inhibition of TSH secretion in this case may be mediated via somatostatin.

Figure 10.2: Structural Formula of TSH

$$\text{PYRO - GLU - HIS - PRO - NH}_2$$

The hormone TRH is a tripeptide originally isolated from extracts of hypothalamus (Figure 10.2). In addition to being found in the hypothalamus, TRH is widely distributed throughout the mammalian brain. Indeed, 70 per cent of the total brain TRH is said to be outside the hypothalamus. Networks of TRH-staining nerve terminals have been observed in several motor nuclei of the brain stem and around motor neurones of the spinal cord, and immunoreactive TRH material has been described in the retina of man and rat. It should be noted that extraneuronal TRH has also been described in the pancreas and gastro-intestinal tract, as well as in the reproductive system and the placenta. TRH is subject to rapid enzymic breakdown in tissues and body fluids. The proglutamyl residue, His-Pro-NH$_2$ is formed, which undergoes cyclicisation to His-Pro-diketopiperazine (DKP). There may also be deamidation of TRH to form TRH free acid. Both these metabolites possess biological activity and can influence the metabolism of TRH. DKP is a potent inhibitor of prolactin release, but the significance of this finding remains uncertain. In addition to stimulating the release of TSH, TRH is a potent stimulus for prolactin secretion in many species, including man. TRH stimulates growth hormone secretion in 60 per cent of patients with acromegaly, as well as in some patients with renal failure, hepatic failure, anorexia nervosa and depressive illness. These responses may be a consequence of changes in GHRH or somatostatin release. Measurement of TRH in the circulation is of little value in studying hypothalamic function because of the wide distribution of the peptide throughout the body, and because of the dilution of portal vessel blood in the systemic circulation and its rapid degradation by proteolytic enzymes.

Binding sites for TRH are found on the plasma membrane of anterior pituitary cells with physiologically-relevant numbers and binding affinities. Evidence that such sites are involved in the TSH or prolactin response is provided by agreement between the relative affinities for binding of TRH analogues and their relative potencies in stimulating hormone release. Despite intensive research over the last few years, knowledge of the intracellular mediation of the action of TSH is fragmentary. In both thyrotrophs and mammotrophs, the response to TRH depends on Ca^{++} but not cyclic AMP, and it seems that an increase in the concentration of free or unbound Ca^{++} in the cytoplasm serves to couple stimulation by TRH to hormone secretion. In mammotrophs, TRH appears to cause a rise in free calcium by a single mechanism, namely mobilisation of cellular calcium. In contrast, in the thyrotrophs, under normal circumstances TRH causes mobilisation of Ca^{++} from a cellular pool (or pools) and also induces a flux of extracellular Ca^{++} through voltage-dependent channels in the plasma membrane.

Many of the established criteria for a neurotransmitter are fulfilled by TRH. It is therefore possible that, in some areas of the central nervous system, TRH functions as an orthodox neurotransmitter, whereas in other areas it modulates the effects of monoamine transmitters. In man it antagonises many effects of opioid peptides (but not the analgesia), elevates blood pressure, and possibly produces psychobiological (antidepressant) effects. It also reduces ataxia in spinocerebellar degeneration, but massive doses are required. Large doses of TRH have also been used in the treatment of shock, in which situation it appears to synergise with naloxone.

Neuropharmacological studies in the rat suggest that TSH secretion is under central α-adrenergic control, but direct studies of TRH from hypothalamic fragments *in vitro* have given contradictory results. Noradrenaline, histamine and serotonin have each been reported to stimulate TRH release. Noradrenaline stimulates TRH release, but there are also α-adrenoceptor binding sites on the thyrotroph. Hypersecretion of TSH in hypothyroid patients can be attenuated through blockade of noradrenaline synthesis. There is also evidence that dopamine exerts an inhibitory influence on TRH release, but the physiological relevance of the dopamine receptor on the thyrotroph is itself controversial. Specific dopamine receptor agonists have been reported to inhibit basal TSH levels and to attenuate TSH release in cold ambient temperatures. Histamine also releases TSH from anterior pituitaries *in vitro*. In contrast, there is no consistent evidence as to the role of serotonergic neurones in TSH regulation, although most data suggests that serotonin inhibits TSH release. Opiates and opioid peptides inhibit the release of TRH in the rat, whereas a small stimulatory effect is seen in man.

Actions of TSH

The primary role of TSH is to regulate differentiated functions in thyroid cells. These include uptake of iodine, thyroglobulin biosynthesis, iodination of thyroglobulin to form the thyroid hormones (T_3 and T_4) and the release of thyroid hormones into the blood stream. Most T_3 is formed by peripheral deiodination of T_4 in the circulation. Another important action of TSH is to stimulate the growth of thyroid cells. This role was suggested by the observation that TSH caused increases in the mitotic index of thyroid glands *in vivo*, and could induce thymidine uptake in primary cultures of thyroid cells or thyroid follicles. It has now been established that growth of a clonal culture of functional thyroid cells is dependent on TSH. Regulation by TSH of differentiated functions and growth must involve a specific cell receptor, either the same or two entirely different molecular entities. Similarly, TSH regulation of differentiated functions and growth may involve the cyclic AMP messenger system, a different signal system such as the Ca^{++} phosphoinositol pathway, or a combination of signals. Studies of the *in vitro* properties of ^{125}I-TSH binding led to the concept that TSH binding to a glycoprotein is the first step in receptor recognition. The full functional response requires a ganglioside intermediary, which may act as an emulsifying agent to allow the hormone to interact with other membrane components.

On stimulation of the thyroid by TSH, a sequence of changes occurs as follows. Initially, there is an increase in cyclic AMP concentrations, somewhat surprisingly an increased efflux of iodide from the cells, increased iodination of thyroglobulin, and colloid droplet formation. It is only then that there is an increased flux of iodide into the cell, with increased hormone release. There is an increase in the number and activity of microvilli and an increase in cell height. Metabolic effects are then seen, with increased carbohydrate turnover (principally via the hexoseshunt pathway, as the thyroid contains little glycogen) and also increased phosholipid turnover. Increased protein synthesis is seen within the cell, especially thyroglobulin, and RNA turnover is enhanced. An important aspect of the TSH response appears to be the effects on the iodide pump, resulting first in an influx of iodide and subsequently in an enhanced efflux. Although the increased metabolic activities, protein-iodination and release of thyroid hormones are observed in response to stimulation by TSH, it does not appear to enhance lysosome activity. The net result of TSH activity is to increase the synthesis and stores of fresh hormone, as well as causing increased release of thyroid hormones. The most recently synthesised thyroglobulin is the first to be removed from the follicle. Since newly-iodinated thyroglobulin surrounding the edge of the follicle has a lower iodine content than the thryoglobulin in the centre, this new thyroglobulin has a relatively high T_3 content. This provides a mechanism for modulating the amounts of T_3 released.

Clinical Syndromes of TSH Dysfunction

TSH Deficiency

In the most common form of hypothyroidism, Hashimoto's thyroiditis, immune-mediated damage to the thyroid produces a fall in circulating T_4 followed by a compensatory rise in serum TSH. In 'subclinical' or 'compensated' hypothyroidism, T_4 then rises to within the normal range. There is little good evidence that this syndrome requires treatment *per se*, but with disease progression the serum T_4 level may become frankly subnormal. In such patients, the elevated TSH level proves the diagnosis of primary hypothyroidism. Occasionally, a borderline fall in T_4 may co-exist with a normal or minimally elevated serum TSH; provocative testing with TRH (200 ug i.v.; sample at 0, 20 and 60 min) will then reveal an exaggerated response as compared with the normal population, again suggesting primary hypothyroidism. A low serum T_4 in the presence of a 'normal' serum TSH suggests pituitary hypothyroidism. TRH testing in these patients is of little use, as such patients may variably have a rise in serum TSH even with pituitary failure. The principal indication for TRH testing in this patient group is to differentiate hypothalamic from pituitary disease: a delayed response to TRH (TSH at 60 min greater than at 20 min) is strongly suggestive of hypothalamic TRH deficiency, although this response is not completely specific.

Absent TSH responses to TRH may be seen in patients with complete TSH deficiency, but such responses are more commonly seen in patients with thyrotoxicosis. In these patients circulating thyroid-stimulating immunoglobulins render the thyroid independent of pituitary control, and the elevated T_3 and T_4 levels block TSH release both basally and in response to TRH. Flat TSH responses to TRH are also seen in some euthyroid patients with ophthalmic Graves' disease or with multinodular goitre, or in the presence of high levels of circulating corticosteroids. Patients with anorexia nervosa, depressive illness and Parkinson's disease may also have an attenuated TSH response to TRH. An exaggerated TSH response to TRH is not infrequently seen in patients with prolactinomas (see Chapter 7).

TSH Excess

Cases of TSH-secreting tumours are extremely rare. In such patients high levels of circulating T_4 and T_3 co-exist with non-suppressed or frankly elevated levels of serum TSH. The tumours are usually large and difficult to treat, requiring surgery and frequently post-operative radiotherapy. Patients with such tumours must be differentiated from patients with functional defects in the regulation of TSH release, in whom there appears to be pituitary resistance to the feedback effects of thyroid hormones. If this defect is restricted to the pituitary, thus altering the set-point about which feedback operates, the patient may be clinically thyrotoxic. However, there may also be generalised resistance to thyroid hormone action, in which case the patient may be euthyroid or even hypothyroid clinically. Patients with a specific pituitary defect in TSH feedback may respond to dopamine agonists or somatostatin, which suppress TSH and thus may inhibit the manifestations of TSH-dependent thyrotoxicosis. Treatment with T_3 may occasionally be useful in suppressing TSH in patients with a specific defect in $T_4 \rightarrow T_3$ conversion. Generally speaking, where the excess TSH is due to adenomatous secretion, there is only poor responsiveness to pharmacological manipulation, although both bromocriptine and somatostatin are worthy of trial. Such tumours are sometimes polymorphous, secreting other pituitary hormones in addition to TSH. A useful diagnostic feature in patients with TSH-secreting tumours is the finding of high circulating levels of α-subunit, the peptide common to the glycoproteins TSH, LH, FSH and hCG. These levels are often much in excess of the complete TSH molecule, and are a strong indicator of adenomatous secretion as opposed to functional defects.

It should be noted that some patients with long-standing primary hypothyroidism may also have enlarged pituitary fossas due to thyrotroph hyperplasia (and possibly hyperprolactinaemia), so that an abnormal fossa in the presence of an elevated serum TSH does not necessarily indicate the presence of a pituitary tumour. Thyrotroph hyperplasia rapidly diminishes in extent with thyroid hormone replacement therapy.

The TRH Test

The details for this test are given in Chapter 14. Patients should be warned that immediately after administration of the TRH they may have a sensation of nausea and of perineal tightening or an urge to micturate. These symptoms are transient. Blood pressure may also rise briefly following TRH, although rarely to high levels. There may have been occasional reports of patients in whom TRH induces an immediate very severe headache, and in some cases this has been associated with pituitary apoplexy. It is not known whether this is secondary to a rise in systemic blood pressure, or is a specific effect of TRH on the tumour vasculature. Patients reporting such symptoms after TRH should not have the test repeated, but fortunately such a reaction is extremely rare.

Further Reading

Chopra, I.J. and Soloman, D.H. (1983) 'Pathogenesis of Hyperthyroidism', *Annual Review of Medicine*, *34*, 267–81

Davies, T.G. (1983) 'Disease of TSH Receptors', *Clinics in Endocrinology and Metabolism, 12*, 79–100

Griffiths, I.C. and Bennet, G.W. (1983) *Thyrotrophin Releasing Hormone*, Raven Press, New York

Jackson, I.M.D. (1982) 'Thyrotrophin Releasing Hormone', *New England Journal of Medicine, 306*, 145–55

Larson P.R. (1982) 'Thyroid-Pituitary Interaction: Feedback Regulation of Thyrotrophin Secretion by Thyroid Hormones', *New England Journal of Medicine 306*, 23–32

Peeters, J.R., Forva, S.M., Dieguez, C. and Scanlon, M.F. (1983) 'TSH Neuroregulation and Alteration in Disease States', *Clinics in Endocrinology and Metabolism 12*, 669–94

11 CORTICOTROPHIN AND ITS RELEASING FACTORS

ACTH and Related Peptides

In the 1930s, many of the anterior pituitary hormones were quite extensively studied but adrenocorticotrophic hormone (ACTH) was relatively neglected. Early in this century it was noticed that damage or removal of the pituitary led to apparent shrinkage of the adrenal glands, but this was attributed to part of the general debilitation. A clear demonstration of the relationship between the pituitary and adrenal came in 1919, when Hofstetter reported a doubling of the adrenal weight of dogs treated with preparations of adenohypophysial extracts. The observations in 1920 of adrenal involution in amphibians lacking a pars distalis, which could be reversed by the administration of fresh anterior-lobe preparations, was entirely overlooked until the observations were reproduced in the rat in 1926. The impure adrenocorticotrophic hormone was isolated by Collip and his team in 1933; 10 years later Li and Evans isolated pure ACTH from sheep pituitaries. The same group described the amino acid sequence of bovine ACTH in 1961. The hormone comprises 39 amino acids and is found in the placenta and hypothalamus as well as the pituitary. The work of the past few years has revealed that ACTH is one of a family of polypeptides co-secreted by the corticotrophs, but is nevertheless the major hormone of physiological significance. The first of the related peptides to be described was β-lipotrophin (i.e.β-LPH), which was isolated in 1965. This was followed by the endorphins and enkephalins. The term 'enkephalin' is derived from the Greek for 'in the head' and refers to the two pentapeptides, met- and leu-enkephalin. Met-enkephalin is included within the 91-residue β-LPH at positions 61 to 65, but it is doubtful whether this particular sequence is ever cleaved from β-LPH on its own. However, a larger peptide running from position 61 to the C-terminus of β-LPH at position 91 is also active at opioid receptors, and is indeed more potent than met-enkephalin as it is more resistant to enzyme degradation. This fragment is termed β-endorphin the related α-endorphin and γ-endorphin are not active at opioid receptors. Unfortunately the word 'endorphin' has also been used to refer to all endogenous opioid peptides, but it should now strictly only be used to refer to these C-terminal derivatives of β-LPH. Whereas β-LPH never appears to yield met-enkephalin, there is good evidence from chromatography that it is partially cleaved in man to release β-endorphin into the circulation. Neither β-LPH itself nor the remaining N-terminal fragment after cleavage (γ-LPH) appear to have any function; the minor lipolytic activity originally described may well have been artefactual. The sequence of β-melanocyte stimulating hormone (β-MSH) is also contained within the residues of β-LPH.

Similarly, ACTH contains the amino acid sequence of α-melanocyte stimulating hormone (α-MSH) and corticotrophin-like intermediate lobe peptide (CLIP). In all species studied, the first 24 amino acids are identical. Minor species differences are found in the C-terminal end of the molecule (that with the free carboxyl group). The first 13 amino acids of ACTH are identical with the MSH molecule of all species, residues 4–10 of MSH being the minimal structural requirements for MSH activity. For this reason β-MSH and ACTH have 22 per cent and 1 per cent of the activity of MSH. Studies of the structure-activity relationships of ACTH indicate that the first 13 amino acids are the minimum required for biological activity. Addition of amino acids 14–20 progressively augments biological activity. Several laboratories have synthesised a peptide consisting of the first 24 amino acids of ACTH 1–39; as this possesses full biological activity, it can be used both diagnostically and therapeutically.

Over the years following the discovery of β-LPH, evidence has been accumulating of a close association with ACTH and, more recently, β-endorphin. For example, concentrations of all three peptides in plasma increase during stress, and immunohistochemical studies have revealed them in the same pituitary cells. It was therefore postulated that synthesis of ACTH and β-LPH was via a common precursor. This has now been identified, and has a molecular weight of 31 000 (hence it is referred to as 31K).

The complete amino acid sequence has been revealed by cloned DNA. The term pro-opiocortin has been coined for this ACTH/LPH precursor. Bovine pro-opiocortin has been demonstrated to contain the sequence of ACTH and β-LPH, which in turn contain respectively the residues of α-MSH and β-MSH. A third MSH sequence termed γ-MSH is found in the N-terminal region, which is now variously referred to as pro-γ-MSH or N-terminal-pro-opiocortin (N-POC). As the polypeptide chain is being synthesised *in vivo*, complex oligosaccharides may be added so that either a protein or α glycosylated protein may be produced, depending on the species, etc. The precursor is cleaved at the site of pairs of basic residues. Pro-opiocortin is found both in the corticotrophs of the anterior pituitary and in the melanotrophs of the intermediate lobe. In the former the precursor yields first a pro-ACTH intermediate (molecular weight 21 000) and β-LPH. This is broken down to release ACTH and pro-γ-MSH into the circulation, whereas β-LPH is partially cleaved to γ-LPH and β-endorphin. Further processing of pro-γ-MSH undoubtedly occurs, but the details are unclear (Figure 11.1A). In summary, pro-opiocortin produces ACTH, β-LPH, and small amounts of β-endorphin and γ-LPH, and there is variable processing of pro-γ-MSH. To complicate the situation further, pro-opiocortin is cleaved quite differently in species that possess a distinct intermediate lobe. Here ACTH is further broken down into α-MSH and CLIP, and the processing of β-LPH is also more complete. However, there is also a process of acetylation, which renders the opioid β-endorphin into opiate-inactive N-acetyl-β-endorphin. With the exception of ACTH, the functions of the members of this diverse series of peptides (Figure 11.1B) are not clear. Nevertheless, there are recent studies which suggest that fragments of pro-γ-MSH may lead to adrenal growth rather than cortisol release, and may potentiate the cortisol-releasing activity of ACTH while being devoid of such intrinsic activity themselves. The initial excitement engendered by finding that an opioid

Figure 11.1A: Processing of Pro-opiocortin in the Anterior Pituitary and Possible Functions of the Peptide Fragments Produced

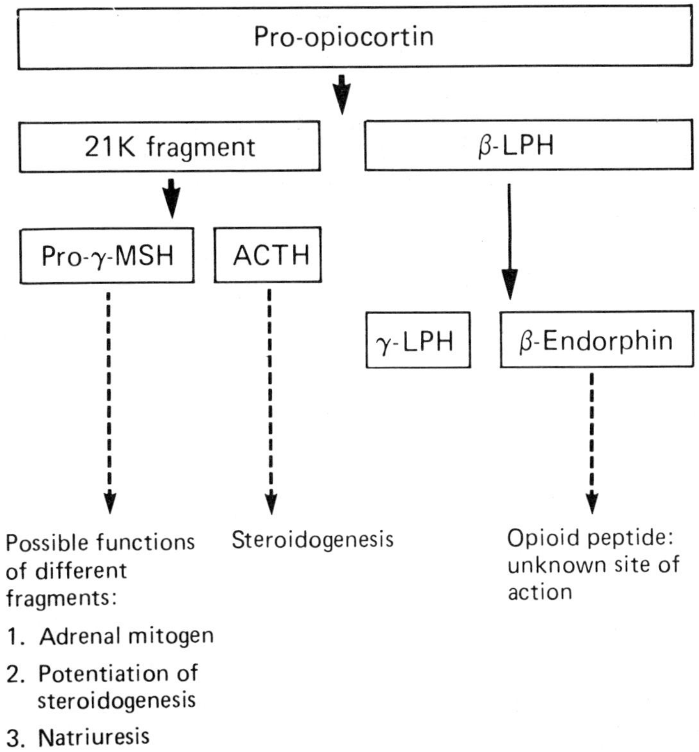

```
                    Pro-opiocortin
                          │
            ┌─────────────┴─────────────┐
            ▼                           ▼
      21K fragment                    β-LPH
            │                           │
      ┌─────┴─────┐                     │
      ▼           ▼                     ▼
  Pro-γ-MSH     ACTH              ┌─────┴─────┐
      ┆           ┆               ▼           ▼
      ┆           ┆             γ-LPH     β-Endorphin
      ┆           ┆               ┆           ┆
      ▼           ▼               ┆           ▼
```

Possible functions of different fragments: Steroidogenesis   Opioid peptide: unknown site of action

1. Adrenal mitogen
2. Potentiation of steroidogenesis
3. Natriuresis

peptide could be released from the pituitary into the general circulation has been dampened by calculations demonstrating extremely low levels of free β-endorphin in the circulation. Pro-opiocortin itself is not released into the blood, but abnormal breakdown products can occur in the case of pituitary or ectopic tumours (see below), or possibly under extreme stimulation.

Production of antisera to the endorphins has allowed studies on the localisation of these peptides throughout the body. In addition to the pituitary gland, they are found throughout the brain and gastro-intestinal tract. Within the pars intermedia they are found in small granules in the cytoplasm. In the anterior pituitary they are found in larger granules in cells surrounding blood vessels. Immunocytochemical studies also indicate that β-endorphin is present in the brain many months after hypophysectomy, which would eliminate the pituitary as a major source.

Assay of ACTH

Many different bioassays have been described for ACTH which are largely

Figure 11.1B: Processing of Pro-opiocortin in the Intermediate Lobe of the Mammalian Pituitary

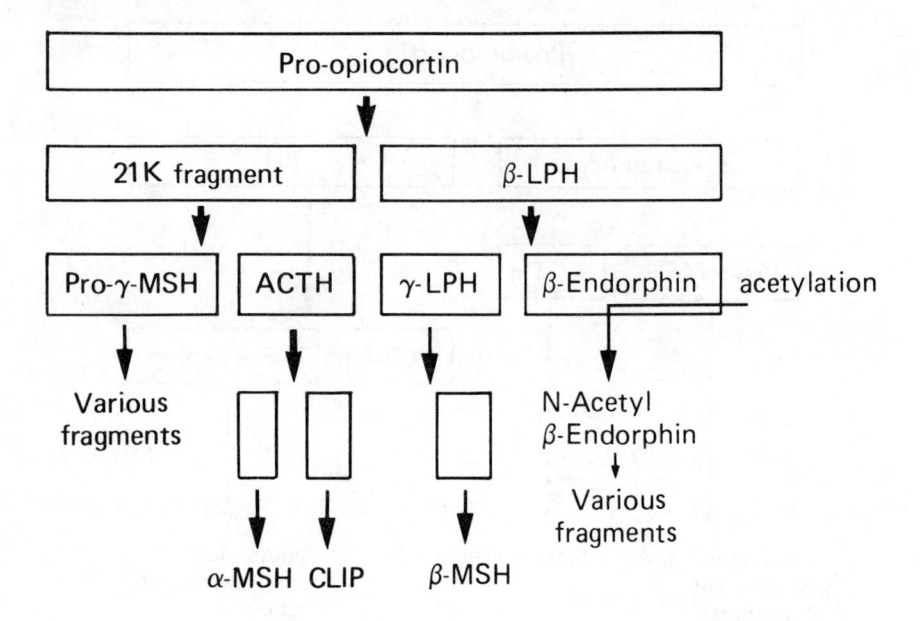

```
                    Pro-opiocortin
                          ↓
        ┌─────────────────┬─────────────────┐
        21K fragment              β-LPH
             ↓                      ↓
    ┌────────┬──────┐        ┌──────┬──────────┐
  Pro-γ-MSH  ACTH            γ-LPH   β-Endorphin    acetylation
     ↓        ↓                ↓         ↓
  Various   ☐  ☐              ☐      N-Acetyl
  fragments                          β-Endorphin
             ↓  ↓              ↓         ↓
           α-MSH CLIP        β-MSH    Various
                                      fragments
```

dependent on the action of the hormone on the adrenal cortex. A number of assays have been described that are sensitive enough to detect circulating concentrations of the hormone, although the throughput is very limited. Early assays depended on ACTH-induced depletion of ascorbic acid in the adrenal gland, or altered steroid metabolism. An *in vivo* bioassay of relatively high sensitivity was the Lipscombe-Nelson bioassay, in which groups of rats were first hypophysectomised to remove the endogenous source of the hormone. Some two hours later, an injection of unknown or standard was given, and 8–10 min later a sample of adrenal venous blood was collected for the determination of cortisol. Since each animal only yields one point for a dose-response curve, relatively large numbers of animals were used and much experimental time was consumed. As indicated in Chapter 3, the cytochemical assay yields a method for ACTH determination that is extremely tedious but is of exquisite sensitivity. It is performed using guinea-pig adrenals, each gland yielding three fragments of tissue for culture. The end-point is the density of staining in the zona reticularis with Prussian blue.

As with most small peptides, establishing a radioimmunoassay did not prove easy. Antisera were difficult to raise and, because of the low circulating concentrations, an extraction step was required. Again, as for most hormones where a bioassay is available, dissociation between biological and immunological activity was demonstrated. Antisera have been raised against the N-terminal and the C-terminal portions of the ACTH molecule, and the use of these and related antisera played a part in establishing the presence of ACTH-related peptides in pituitary and blood samples. Thus, assays employing antisera against the

C-terminal region of β-LPH will detect both β-LPH and β-endorphin, and N-terminal assays detect both β- and γ-LPH. An excess of C-terminal as opposed to N-terminal LPH immunoreactivity is suggestive of the presence of excess β-endorphin. Similarly, most ACTH assays will not distinguish between 'free' ACTH or ACTH still combined with pro-γ-MSH. This latter species, which is not normally present but can occur in patients with ACTH-secreting tumours, is 'big ACTH'. As this form does not have the same biological activity as free ACTH, there will obviously be a notable discrepancy between ACTH bioactivity and immunoreactivity. It is likely that the immunoradiometric assays in which antibodies react with both ends of ACTH (see Chapter 3) will also differentiate free ACTH from its precursor molecule(s).

In general, whatever the type of assay for ACTH, there are a number of points that must be taken into consideration. The release of ACTH is episodic, and also shows a circadian rhythm, so it is important that blood sampling is always performed at the same time of the day. It should also be borne in mind that ACTH is a stress-released hormone. Furthermore, it is rapidly broken down in plasma so that samples should be cooled on collection and spun in a cool centrifuge, and the plasma immediately separated and then rapidly deep-frozen. In addition, since ACTH is adsorbed onto glass, plastic containers should be used throughout.

Control of ACTH Secretion

ACTH secretion is largely controlled by the hypothalamus, so in considering release of this trophic hormone one is essentially considering the release of CRF. For the sake of simplicity the control of ACTH secretion may be said to be exerted through three principal mechanisms, the negative feedback of glucocorticoids, circadian rhythm and stress. Similiar stimuli influence the release of the ACTH-related peptides in man such as pro-γ-MSH, β-LPH and β-endorphin.

Corticotrophin Releasing Factor

There was a delay of more than 25 years between the discovery of CRF and its chemical characterisation. Many naturally occurring substances, such as the neurohypophysial hormones, catecholamines and angiotensin II, were known to have ACTH stimulating properties, but none had the full spectrum of activity for a CRF. Isolation was impeded by a number of factors, including problems with assays for the factor, the tiny quantities present in the brain, and the fact that CRF had an unexpectedly high molecular weight close to that of ACTH, leading to problems with gel filtration. Isolation of CRF was achieved by Vale and his colleagues working with the aqueous phase of an extract of about half a million sheep hypothalami. Ovine CRF was found to be a 41-residue, straight-chain, terminally amidated peptide, homologous with several known peptides, including sauvagine (isolated from frog skin), urotensin I (isolated from the urohypophysis of some fish), calmodulin and angiotensinogen. This peptide will be referred to as CRF-41 (Figure 11.2). Human CRF has recently been sequenced;

140 Corticotrophin and its Releasing Factors

Figure 11.2: The Structure of Ovine CRF

H—Ser—Gln—Glu—Pro—Pro—Ile—Ser—Leu—Asp—Leu—Thr—

Phe—His—Leu—Leu—Arg—Glu—Val—Leu—Gle—Met—Thr—Lys—

Ala—Asp—Gln—Leu—Ala—Gln—Gln—Ala—His—Ser—Asn—Arg—

Lys—Leu—Leu—Asp—Ile—Ala—NH$_2$

it is identical to rat CRF, but differs by seven amino acids from ovine CRF.

Distribution of CRF within the hypothalamus has been mapped. It is found in the mediobasal region, the cell bodies lying predominantly in the parvicellular parts of the paraventricular nucleus. Immunostaining is also found in the paraventricular nucleus in the monkey and the supraoptic nucleus of the sheep, and in the vicinity of the basal hypothalamic cells which contain pro-opiomelanocortin derivatives. Physiologically significant levels of CRF have been demonstrated in portal blood. Ovine CRF-41 is highly effective in stimulating ACTH and cortisol release in man (Figure 11.3).

In addition to the paraventricular-infundibular pathway, CRF has been found in experimental animals in other areas of the central nervous systems. One major region is that known to regulate the autonomic nervous system; another consists of interneurones in the cerebral cortex. Thus it is possible that CRF may also play a role in neuroendocrine regulation, possibly modulating the output of the autonomic nervous system and being involved in cortical integrative mechanisms. There are also explant results showing that CRF produces EEG arousal, general behavioural activation and increased sensitivity to stress. Hence CRF may play a role in a basic and fundamental activating system which would allow the organism not only to mobilise the pituitary-adrenal system in response to an environmental challenge, but also to modulate the central nervous system.

Although vasopressin is no longer a candidate as the most important CRF, none the less it appears to play a role in the control of ACTH secretion. Vasopressin greatly potentiates the ACTH-releasing activity of CRF-41, both in rat and man, and studies with specific antisera suggest that both peptides are involved in the physiological release of ACTH (although CRF-41 is probably the more important). There are also data showing that CRF-41 and vasopressin may co-exist in hypothalamic neurones, possibly as part of a large ACTH-releasing complex. Angiotensin II may also be part of the complex, although both it and vasopressin can in addition probably modulate the release of CRF-41. An interaction between CRF and catecholamines is also observed, and this appears to be of particular significance with regard to stress. Attempts have been made to characterise the neurotransmitters of the neurone groups affecting the CRF-producing neurones. Many difficulties have been encountered, possibly because the influence of neurotransmitters may depend on the existing background

Figure 11.3: The Effect of 100 μg Ovine CRF (i.v.) on plasma ACTH and cortisol in six normal males. (Reproduced from Grossman *et al.*, 1981, by permission of the authors, and of the Editor of the *Lancet*.)

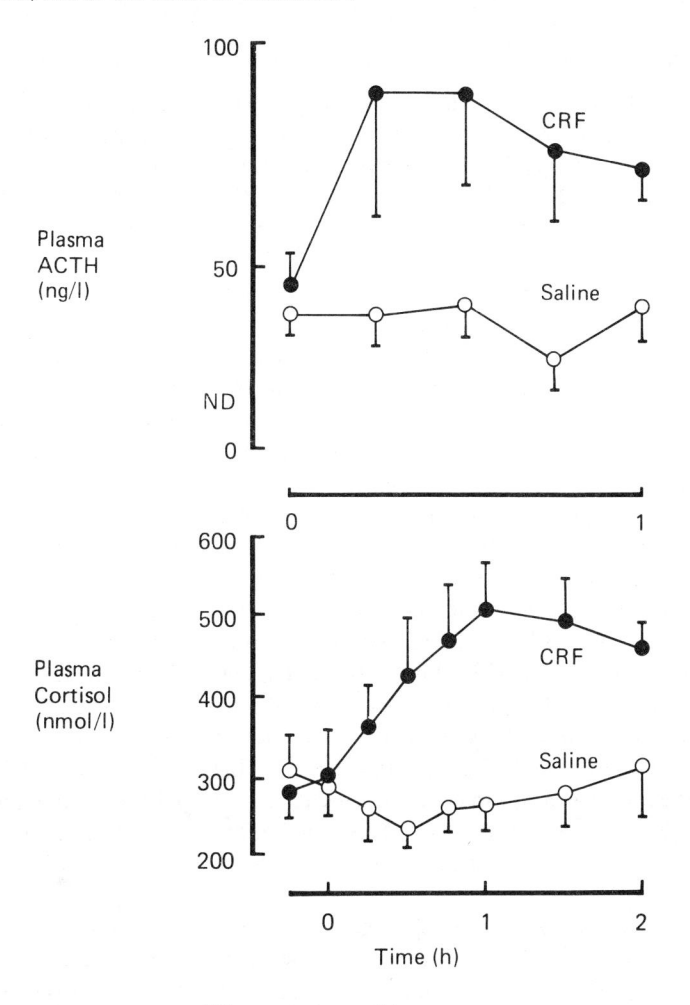

ND = not detectable

conditions imposed by circadian rhythms, etc. Acetylcholine, serotonin and histamine appear to be stimulatory whereas GABA is inhibitory. There is considerable controversy about the role of noradrenaline in the release of CRF in the rat, with evidence for both stimulatory and inhibitory action. However, in man the limited information available suggests a predominantly stimulatory role. Opioid peptides inhibit ACTH release in man through naloxone-insensitive receptors.

As with other peptide hormones, the action of CRF on the pituitary cells probably involves the interaction with plasma membrane receptors giving rise to an increase in cyclic AMP. Secretion of ACTH due to CRF is also calcium dependent. In addition to short term release of ACTH, CRF can lead to increased hormone synthesis.

Feedback Regulation

It was shown in 1938 that administration of extracts of adrenal cortex to rats resulted in hypoplasia of the adrenal glands, suggesting that corticosteroids suppress the secretion of ACTH which otherwise would enhance growth and metabolic action of the target glands. Cortisol, the corticosteroid secreted in the greatest quantity by the human adrenal (some 15 mg per day), exerts a negative feedback effect such that a reciprocal relationship exists between ACTH and cortisol. Following adrenalectomy, or in conditions where there is an enzyme deficiency resulting in a fall in circulating cortisol, the concentration of ACTH is elevated. There is some controversy as to the major site of cortisol action in this regard, i.e., whether it acts principally at the level of the hypothalamus or of the pituitary. However, it does appear to inhibit both the adenohypophysial response to CRF as well as inhibiting secretion of CRF by hypothalamic neurones. Certainly, cortisol receptors are found in both the brain and the pituitary. The concentrations of glucocorticoid receptors in the central nervous system increase during development and after adrenalectomy, whereas those in the pituitary are unaffected. In man, dexamethasone suppresses the pituitary corticotroph response to CRF-41. In addition, data from animals indicate that at both sites there is rate-responsive feedback, and it is possible to divide corticosteroid feedback further into short-term and long-term effects (see below). Cortisol circulates in the blood in association with a binding protein, transcortin or cortisol binding globulin (CBG). The free fraction alone produces biological activity and it is this fraction that is important in the feedback mechanism. Interestingly, the pituitary contains large amounts of a transcortin-like material which seems to be tightly bound to pituitary cells or is present within the cytosol. This material has been proposed to act as a buffer, binding endogenous glucocorticoids and thus diminishing binding to the cortisol receptors.

The results of studies in both experimental animals and man suggest that the feedback of cortisol on ACTH release exhibits two phases. The fast phase occurs immediately after steroid administration, and the second, slow phase is seen some hours later. The fast feedback seems to be related to the rate of increase in circulating corticosteroids, whereas the delayed feedback is dose-related. During this second period of delayed feedback, stress is unable to increase ACTH release. This delayed response can be blocked by administration of a protein synthesis inhibitor. There also appear to be different structural requirements of the glucocorticoid for fast and delayed feedback. The feedback effect of cortisol is termed the 'long-loop' feedback. ACTH is also believed to feed back at the level of the hypothalamus to control its own secretion. This is termed 'short-loop' feedback. The elevation of hypothalamic CRF seen after adrenalectomy indicates that the action of glucocorticoids on ACTH could in part be mediated through changes in CRF secretion. Glucocorticoids have been clearly demonstrated to modulate the response of the pituitary cells to CRF-41 or other secretagogues *in vitro*. It is of note that, even in the presence of very high doses of dexamethasone, CRF-41 can elicit some degree of ACTH secretion, and in man, stress-induced release of CRF-41 can also overcome feedback inhibition if the stimulus is strong enough.

Circadian Rhythm

The rate of ACTH secretion, in common with other pituitary hormones, is not constant throughout the day, but exhibits a number of secretory episodes superimposed on a 24-h periodicity which is a function of the sleep-wake cycle. Peak secretion is seen between 07.00 and 08.00 with a subsequent progressive fall until, at midnight and in the early morning hours, secretion is at a minimum. Cortisol secretion exhibits a virtually identical pattern. Althouth light can cause ACTH secretion to increase, this pattern of secretion is still seen in the blind, and in subjects maintained in constant light or dark, but becomes entrained to a new sleep-wake pattern after about 7 days, for example in shift workers or following intercontinental travel. The pattern also persists after adrenalectomy and during prolonged sleeplessness and bed rest. By the age of three years in the human, this circadian rhythm is established and is maintained throughout life. It could arise from cyclical changes in the neurones sensitive to cortisol or in the activity of neurones controlling CRF secretion.

Stress-induced Release

Many stresses, both physiological and psychological, result in rapid elevation of circulating ACTH concentrations. These include pain, surgery, hypoglycaemia, fever, fear and noise. This effect of the central nervous system on ACTH secretion is not modulated by changes in plasma cortisol concentrations, and can override the feedback control and changes associated with the sleep-wake cycle.

Plasma Concentration of ACTH

In normal healthy individuals, ACTH concentrations in plasma at 08.00 - 10.00 range between 10 and 70 pg/ml, falling to below 10 pg/ml at midnight. ACTH disappears rapidly from the plasma, with a half-time of approximately 20 min. Studies on clearance rates allow determination of the daily secretion rate, which is in the region of 5–20 μg/24 h; a relatively small fraction of the total pituitary content of 250 μg is secreted each day.

Actions of ACTH

The main action of ACTH, and probably the only one of physiological significance, is on the adrenal cortex. This aspect of the physiology of the hormone is covered in greater detail in the volume on steroid hormones, but a brief account will be given here. The adrenal effects of ACTH include increased blood flow, a rapid decrease in cholesterol concentration associated with an increased content of several steroids, and a fall in the ascorbic acid content. There is increased protein synthesis and, if the stimulation is prolonged, adrenal hyperplasia. Of the three zones of the adrenal cortex (the zona glomerulosa, the zona fasciculata and the zona reticularis), ACTH controls the development of the inner two zones, the zona fasciculata and reticularis. These two zones, which secrete steroids with predominantly glucocorticoid activity, hypertrophy on treatment with ACTH, which augments the synthesis of both protein and RNA. However, recent studies have indicated that it is a peptide (or peptides) co-secreted with ACTH that may be the principal stimulant of adrenal growth. Steroids are not stored within the adrenal cortex, but are synthesised immediately prior to release. The precursor of all steroid molecules is cholesterol, which has a long side-chain and lacks the particular configuration which is essential for the activity of steroids. In the synthesis of steroids the cholesterol side-chain is first cleaved and a ketone group introduced, under the control of cholesterol desmolase, to form pregnenolone. The Δ^4–3–one configuration is then introduced to form the biologically active progesterone. By substitution of various side-groups, the many steroids produced by the adrenal cortex are formed. ACTH controls the initial step under the influence of cholesterol desmolase. The first step in ACTH action is binding to specific receptors in the plasma membrane, as described in Chapter 6, which results in the formation of cyclic AMP and the production of a protein kinase. The subsequent steps are unknown, but it has been suggested that there is activation of the phosphorylases necessary for the formation of NADPH, which in turn is required for steroidogenesis. Alternatively, there could be synthesis of an as yet unknown protein which could aid in the many steps associated with the formation of pregnenolone from cholesterol, namely, penetration of cholesterol into the mitochondria, formation of ribosomal proteins or of enzymes, and exit of pregnenolone from the mitochondria. ACTH has a number of extra-adrenal activities, general metabolic effects including an adipolytic effect, melanocyte stimulation and behavioural effects. Of these, the ones exciting most interest at present, and which may prove of significance in the future, are the possible effects on learning. As yet this has only been demonstrated on experimental animals, but molecules containing the sequence of amino acids 4–10 of ACTH have been shown to influence learning and behaviour. At present, the only extra-adrenal effect of clinical significance is the melanocyte-stimulating activity that causes the pigmentation seen in some patients with, for example, Nelson's syndrome.

Over-production of ACTH

Long-term overproduction of cortisol produces the clinical features collectively termed Cushing's syndrome. That form of the disease caused by excessive secretion of ACTH by the pituitary is termed Cushing's disease. It arises from disturbance of the pituitary-hypothalamic mechanisms controlling ACTH release. Increased circulating concentrations of ACTH also result from a fall in plasma cortisol, which may be seen in adrenal failure, or from ectopic production by a tumour. As cortisol in man is solely controlled by ACTH, it provides a useful marker of corticotroph activity. Its half-life of c. 90 minutes is considerably longer than that of ACTH and it has greater stability; it is therefore a useful and reliable guide to integrated ACTH activity over a period of time. The cortisol assay is also considerably easier than for ACTH. Until recently the standard assay technique has been by fluorimetry, although this has had several important disadvantages. In the first place relatively large volumes of blood are required, which are subject to an extraction procedure. In addition, several drugs also fluoresce in this assay, most notably spironolactone and the metabolites of the anti-androgen cyproterone acetate. Furthermore, high levels of endogenous lipids interfere with the assay, and tumours secreting more highly fluorescent compounds such as corticosterone will falsely elevate plasma 'cortisol'. For this reason most laboratories now use a radioimmunoassay for cortisol, which uses small volumes of plasma or serum and can produce very reliable results. However, it should be noted that some steroid compounds such as the endogenous 11–deoxycortisol (the immediate precursor of cortisol) may also cross-react to some extent with this assay, as may drugs such as prednisolone.

Underproduction of ACTH

It is very rare to see underproduction of ACTH as an isolated deficiency. Usually it occurs in association with growth hormone and gonadotrophin deficiency, and frequently also with TSH deficiency. ACTH deficiency results in decreased production of cortisol and adrenal androgens so that the patient exhibits weakness, hypoglycaemia and weight loss. Isolated ACTH deficiency may be associated with excess alcohol intake. Analysis of CRF tests in patients with isolated ACTH deficiency has demonstrated that the majority are indeed deficient in ACTH. However, there is at least one recorded case of such a patient responding to CRF-41 with a rise in ACTH, so that the disorder was in CRF production or release.

Cushing's Disease

Cushing's syndrome refers to the clinical or biochemical manifestations of glucocorticoid cold excess: in Cushing's disease this is due to the abnormal production of ACTH by the pituitary, a clearer term probably being 'pituitary-dependent Cushing's syndrome'. The cause of pituitary-dependent Cushing's syndrome is usually a pituitary basophil adenoma, although very occasionally basophil hyperplasia is seen.

Pituitary-dependent Cushing's syndrome may affect any age group, and has a higher incidence in women. Its clinical manifestations are well known. Glucocorticoid excess causes protein catabolism, and hence thin skin and muscle weakness-'steroid myopathy'. The protein breakdown probably also accounts for the osteoporosis usually seen. Changes in lipolysis are reflected in centripetal obesity, facial mooning and the 'buffalo hump'. Cortisol is diabetogenic, but although glucose intolerance is common, diabetes mellitus is only seen in the more severe cases. Capillary fragility and the thin skin produce the characteristic easy bruising, and the latter in the presence of central obesity (and probably elevated ACTH) gives rise to purple abdominal striae. Adrenal hypersecretion of androgens may produce acne and a greasy skin (seborrhoea), excess facial and body hair (hirsuties), and menstrual irregularity (oligmenorrhoea) in women, with the secondary development of polycystic ovaries. Renal calculi are not infrequent, and there is immunosuppression so that fungal skin infections with candidiasis or pityriasis versicolor occur very commonly. Hypertension is due to the mineralocorticoid effects of cortisol, aldosterone production being normal or reduced; hypokalaemia is very rare in the absence of diuretic therapy.

The primary abnormality appears to be in the secretion of ACTH, which loses its circadian pattern and is unresponsive to stress. Steroid feedback becomes less effective but does not disappear. These phenomena provide the biochemical basis of the biochemical tests for pituitary-dependent Cushing's syndrome. Thus the absence of circadian rhythmicity is indicated by a cortisol concentration above 180 nmol/litre in a serum sample taken at midnight from a sleeping patient (the patient should be well hospitalised and asleep, or stress-induced rises vitiate the test). It should be noted that the 9 a.m. serum cortisol may well be normal in patients with only mild disease. Total urinary free cortisol is usually elevated, however, and even the relatively crude estimate of urinary 17-hydroxycorticosteroids may be useful diagnostically if it is related to the urinary creatinine. During the stress of insulin-induced hypoglycaemia, serum cortisol fails to rise in at least 80 per cent of cases. Following low-dose dexamethasone (0.5 mg six-hourly for 48 h), urinary cortisol metabolites (11-hydroxycorticosteroids) are markedly suppressed in normal subjects, and at the end of the test taken at 9 a.m. serum cortisol is below 200 nmol/litre; little or no fall is seen in any form of Cushing's syndrome. However, the *relative* insensitivity is revealed in pituitary-dependent Cushing's syndrome by the suppression of urinary 11-hydroxycorticosteroids (>50 per cent) and serum cortisol (>200 nmol/litre) following high-dose dexamethasone (2 mg six-hourly for 48 h). A useful out-patient screening test for Cushing's syndrome is to administer 1 mg dexamethasone at 11 p.m. to midnight, and measure serum cortisol the next morning at 8–9 a.m. A serum cortisol below 180 nmol/litre almost totally excludes Cushing's syndrome. False positives do occur, so more extensive tests are required in the patients failing to show suppression. In patients with the ectopic ACTH syndrome or an adrenal tumour, such suppression is not seen, although it is not possible to make the differentiation in all cases. Plasma ACTH is only useful in detecting patients with an adrenal adenoma or carcinoma (when it is undetectable) or in identifying the most obvious cases of the ectopic ACTH syndrome (when it is grossly elevated). Almost all patients with pituitary-dependent Cushing's syndrome have plasma ACTH levels that are either within the normal range or are only moderately elevated.

Patients with pituitary-dependent Cushing's syndrome must be differentiated

Table 11.1: Diagnosis of Cushing's Syndrome

Test	Comments
Absent circadian rhythm of cortisol	Night sample must be taken asleep. Rhythm may be absent in depressive illness
Failure of plasma cortisol to suppress (180 nmol/litre at 09.00) with low dose dexamethasone 0.5 mg 6-hourly x 8	Failure to suppress may also be present in depressive illness or marked obesity
Failure of plasma cortisol to rise during insulin-induced hypoglycaemia	May require high dose of insulin, e.g. 0.3 U/kg. Probably highly sensitive and specific, but little published data. Criterion of 'response' not clearly defined
Urinary excretion of:	
17-ketogenic steroids	Little use
17-ketosteroids	Little use
11-OH-corticosteroids	Sensitive test, especially when corrected for urinary creatinine. May also be elevated in depressive illness and obesity
CRF-41: 100 μg or 1 μg/kg i.v.	Precise data needed, but an exuberant response with plasma cortisol increasing to beyond 1000 mmol/litre suggests Cushing's disease
Differential diagnosis: Biochemical tests	
Plasma ACTH at 09.00	Very low or undetectable = adrenal tumour. Normal range or slightly elevated = Cushing's disease or ectopic ACTH. Very high = ectopic ACTH
Failure of urinary hydrocortiscosteroids or plasma cortisol to suppress by 50% on high-dose dexamethasone 2 mg 6-hourly x 8	Ectopic ACTH or adrenal tumour; small incidence of false positives and false negatives
Failure of 17-ketogenic steroids to double on day of, or day following, metyrapone 750 mg 4 hourly x 6	Ectopic ACTH or adrenal tumour. Patient needs hospitalisation. Very poor reliability, although a serum 11-deoxycortisol level of less than 1000 mmOl/litre at 24 h suggestive of non-pituitary disease
CRF-41: 100 μg or 1 μg/kg i.v.	Absent response strongly suggests adrenal tumour or ectopic ACTH
Plasma K$^+$	Hypokalaemia usually indicative of non-pituitary disease
Radiological Procedures	
Sampling of great veins for ACTH	Petrosal sinus sampling with simultaneous peripheral sample most useful for confirming Cushing's disease. Caution needs to be taken as ACTH is a pulsatile hormone
High-resolution CT scan	Good for localising 1. large adrenal tumours; 2. ectopic sources; 3. large pituitary tumours. Small pituitary tumours or ectopic sources may escape detection
Ultrasound	Rarely helpful except for pancreatic ectopic sources in thin patients
Adrenal scintigraphy	Rarely helpful: high unilateral uptake suggests adrenal adenoma. Adrenal carcinoma has poor uptake

from patients with obesity and depressive illnesses, as in both of these circadian rhythmicity may be lost and there may also be partial resistance to dexamethasone. This is particularly relevant in the case of depressive illness, as two-thirds of patients with Cushing's disease have overt psychiatric disease and in one-third it may be florid and even manifest itself as a psychosis. There is also the syndrome of so-called alcoholic 'pseudo-Cushing's', in which excess alcohol intake is associated with a number of clinical and biochemical features of Cushing's syndrome. The disorder is, by its nature, evanescent, as hospitalisation almost invariably leads to the cessation of alcohol intake. Indeed, some authorities even question its existence as they consider that the transient biochemical features suggestive of Cushing's syndrome merely reflect the stress of alcohol withdrawal.

More difficult is the differential diagnosis between pituitary-dependent Cushing's syndrome and the ectopic ACTH syndrome. The latter may be less rare than previously thought, and patients need not have the gross hyperpigmentation which is seen, for example, in patients with oat-cell carcinomas of the bronchus. Blockade of the final biosynthetic step in cortisol production (11-deoxycortisol→cortisol; compound 'S'→compound 'F') with metyrapone (750 mg four-hourly for 6 h) leads to a rapid fall in cortisol in all patients; in normal subjects there is a compensatory rise in ACTH such that the urinary precursor metabolites of cortisol (17-ketogenic steroids) are elevated on the day *of*, or the day *following*, metyrapone administration. Classically, this response is exaggerated in Cushing's syndrome (urinary steroids rise > 100 per cent) and absent in the ectopic ACTH syndrome (Figure 11.4). Unfortunately, the discriminatory power of this test is poor. However, recent data suggest that measuring serum 11-deoxycortisol at the completion of the test (+24 h) may be a much better discriminator, with levels above 1000 nmol/litre strongly suggestive of pituitary-dependent Cushing's syndrome. It has been suggested that stimulation with CRF-41 may be useful diagnostically with an excessive response in Cushing's disease and little or no response in the ectopic ACTH syndrome. Again, unfortunately, this clear distinction is only seen in the most obvious cases.

Other biochemical changes are common to all forms of glucocorticoid excess. The growth hormone response to hypoglycaemia is usually blunted or absent (and is one cause of poor growth in childhood Cushing's); there is a poor TSH response to TRH; and gonadotrophins may be partially suppressed. Sex hormone binding globulin (SHBG) is considerably reduced, further increasing the already elevated levels of adrenal androgens in women. Interestingly, hypokalaemia, which is very strongly correlated with the ectopic ACTH syndrome, is rare in Cushing's disease unless the pituitary tumour is large and invasive. Precursor forms of ACTH — 'big ACTH' — are also often seen in the ectopic ACTH syndrome and may be demonstrated by chromatography or, more elegantly, by a discrepancy in ACTH measured by conventional RIA and immunoradiometric assay (see Chapter 3) or bioassay. Again, 'big ACTH' can be present in patients with Cushing's syndrome and very large pituitary tumours, and it has been suggested that the coupling of pro-γ-MSH and ACTH in the usual form of 'big ACTH' in some way potentiates adrenal adrenocorticoid production and hence hypokalaemia.

Figure 11.4: In Normal Subjects There Is a Feedback Regulation of ACTH and Cortisol Release (A). Following Blockade of Cortisol Synthesis with Metyrapone, There Is an Increase in ACTH and Cortisol Precursors in Normals and an Enhanced Release in Pituitary-dependent Cushing's Syndrome (B); in the Ectopic ACTH Syndrome, no Increase in ACTH and Precursors is seen (C)

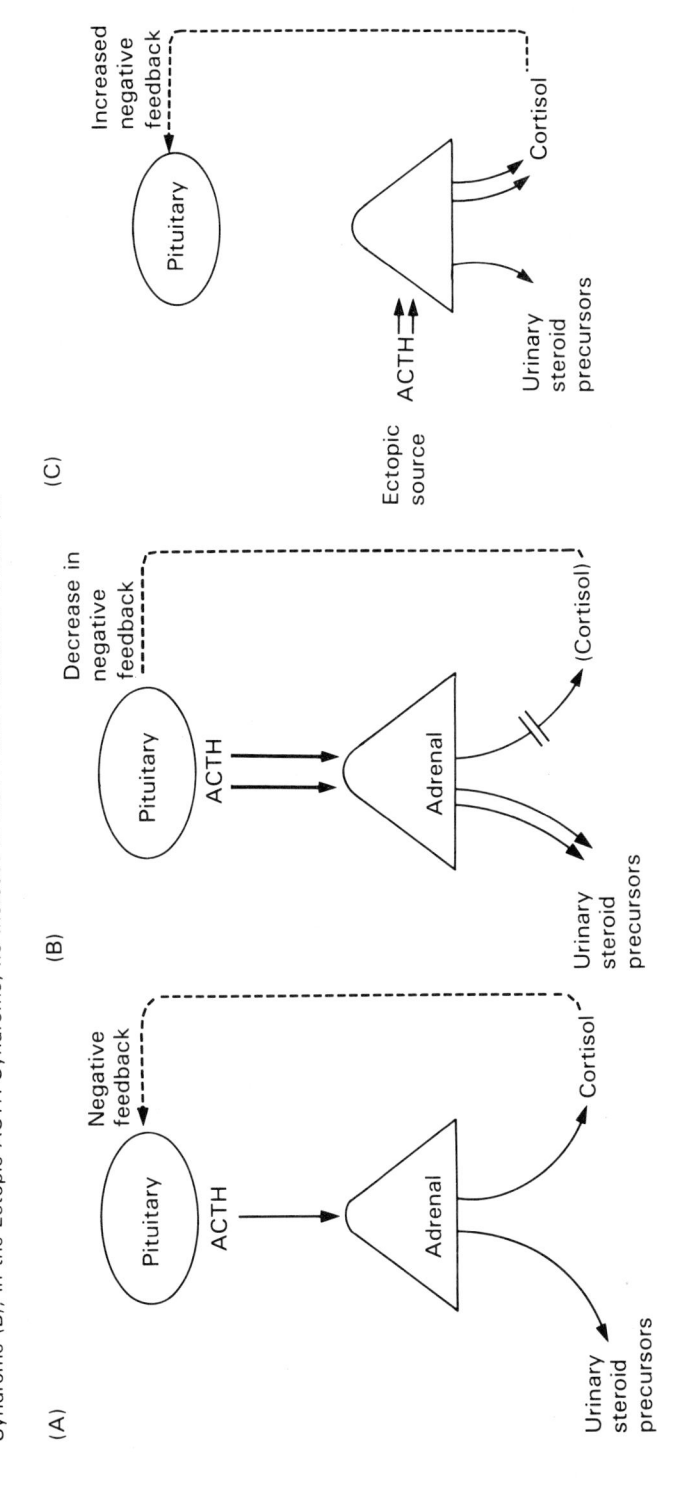

Hyperprolactinaemia is seen is some 40 per cent of patients in both the ectopic ACTH syndrome and pituitary-dependent Cushing's syndrome.

Treatment

Treatment of Cushing's disease is aimed both at lowering the excess cortisol production and at controlling the pituitary tumour. Blockade of cortisol secretion with the 11-hydroxylase inhibitor metyrapone will usually cause a 'medical adrenalectomy' and is important first-line management in almost all cases. The patient rapidly improves symptomatically, and the fall in cortisol is often accompanied by a characteristic desquamation of the skin. When the daily production rate of cortisol is within the normal range, usually at a time that the mean cortisol is 300-400 nmol/litre, more definitive treatment can be undertaken. Although 80 to 90 per cent of such patients have a normal pituitary fossa on plain skull radiology, basophil microadenomas are harboured by the pituitary in almost all of these cases. These may be revealed as hypodense or isodense lesions on high-resolution CT scanning. Surgical adrenalectomy and cortisol replacement removes part of the steroid feedback to these tumours, and Nelson's syndrome (enlarging pituitary tumour, pigmentation, and very high levels of ACTH) will develop in at least 20 to 30 per cent of such patients. Megavoltage radiotherapy by a linear accelerator considerably decreases the incidence of Nelson's syndrome. It has the advantage that the mean serum cortisol production will fall progressively until the patient can be weaned off metyrapone altogether, although in many patients this may take several years. Yttrium implantation radiotherapy is similar but acts more rapidly; however, it is only available in very few centres. Microadenomectomy by the trans-sphenoidal approach can produce an immediate cure in the majority (70–90 per cent) of patients, and in good hands the residual pituitary function remains intact (apart from occasional perioperative diabetes insipidus). The tumours are usually small and centrally located, and can be stained with ACTH-antiserum. The remaining normal corticotrophs also show Crooke's change, i.e. they have a hyaline atrophic appearance due to neurofilamentous accumulation. Thus, successful adenomectomy is immediately followed by an absence of ACTH and cortisol secretion, and patients will need to be on hydrocortisone replacement therapy until their own pituitary-adrenal axis recovers. This may take up to 18 months or occasionally longer. Large tumours should probably additionally have postoperative radiotherapy. Trans-sphenoidal surgery is probably the initial treatment of choice for Cushing's disease.

Other medical agents that will block cortisol biosynthesis include aminoglutethimide, trilostane, and o'p'DDD (Mitotane). Aminoglutethimide has a high incidence of nausea and rashes associated with its use and is rarely totally effective on its own; experience with trilostane has also not been favourable. Early studies suggested that o'p'DDD, which is related to DDT and is adrenolytic, also caused unacceptable side-effects, particularly nausea and ataxia, but more recent work indicates that these are associated with toxic impurities, and that total daily doses of the purified o'p'DDD alone can be well tolerated. As the drug is adrenotoxic and steadily accumulates, some French groups have claimed that treatment with o'p'DDD alone can eventually cure Cushing's disease. Etomidate is a new anaesthetic that blocks cortisol biosynthesis but is unlikely to be useful clinically in this context.

Patients with the ectopic ACTH syndrome should be treated with metyrapone in the first instance, followed by removal of the source of the ACTH — usually a carcinoid tumour of the bronchus, thymus or pancreas. The tumour may be localised by whole-body CT scanning, or possibly by selective sampling for ACTH by a venous catheter which may reveal even very small tumours. Occasionally, no tumour can be located, in which case metyrapone therapy and regular review are necessary. It is important to note that in both forms of Cushing's syndrome there may be a cyclicity of ACTH release, with a periodic waxing and waning occurring over days, weeks or months. This may make control with metyrapone difficult.

Very occasionally, neurotransmitter drugs may directly alter the secretion of ACTH by pituitary microadenomas. Bromocriptine is sometimes effective, although in our experience the great majority of patients do not respond. It has been suggested that in patients responding to bromocriptine, the tumour arises from the pars intermedia. Such patients are also resistant to high-dose dexamethasone. However, the evidence for this theory is unconvincing. An alternative medical therapy is provided by the serotonin antagonist cyproheptadine. The rationale for this treatment is blockade of serotonin-mediated CRF release. However, as cyproheptadine directly suppresses ACTH release *in vitro* from pituitary tumour cells taken from responsive patients, it seems more likely that the action of cyproheptadine is unrelated to its neurotransmitter properties. The high incidence of sedation and excessively increased appetite with this drug renders it less useful clinically than had been originally supposed. Finally, recent studies have indicated that sodium valproate, which elevates central GABA levels, can lower ACTH levels in some patients with Nelson's syndrome and pituitary-dependent Cushing's syndrome. These findings have not been confirmed and await re-evaluation. In general, neuropharmacological therapy is best reserved for those patients with resistant tumours that have defied surgical and radiotherapeutic procedures.

In summary, it would be reasonable to submit patients with Cushing's disease to selective adenomectomy if local expertise is available. If this is not available, or if operation is unsuccessful, radiotherapy with interim metyrapone therapy is a reasonable alternative, current data indicating the prospect of long-term cure in at least 50 per cent of patients. Bilateral adrenalectomy should probably be reserved for patients intolerant of metyrapone who wish to conceive, or in whom cyclicity renders metyrapone control difficult. It should always be accompanied by radiotherapy. Neurotransmitter therapy may be useful in patients with large tumours resistant to surgery and radiotherapy.

Aetiology

A small but not insignificant minority of patients with pituitary-dependent Cushing's syndrome have pituitary corticotroph hyperplasia. In such patients it is possible that there is an increase in endogenous CRF release. One could speculate that such CRF overproduction is fundamental to all patients with Cushing's disease, but that in the majority this eventually leads to the development of an autonomous adenoma. It has been reported that patients with Cushing's disease have EEG abnormalities not seen in other forms of Cushing's syndrome, suggestive of a central CNS abnormality. However, proof for this theory depends on the long-term rate of recurrence of 'cured' patients treated by hypophysectomy, as well as the discriminative use of the new CRF assays. Occasional patients have been described with the 'ectopic ACTH' syndrome and pituitary corticotroph hyperplasia, suggesting the presence of ectopic CRF which secondarily stimulates the pituitary. These CRFs have rarely been analysed biochemically, but in at least one reported case the 'CRF' was related to the amphibian skin peptide bombesin. Tumours arising from the residual pars intermedia are probably less common than originally reported, but may represent the small subgroup who are dopamine-sensitive and more dexamethasone-resistant than usual.

Further Reading

Bloom, F.E. (1983) 'Endorphins: a Growing Family of Pharmacologically Prominent Peptides', *Annual Review of Pharmacology and Toxicology, 23* 151-70

Gillies, G. and Grossman, A. (1985) 'The CRFs and their Control: Chemistry, Physiology and Clinical Implications', *Clinics in Endocrinology and Metabolism, 14,* in press

Howlett, T.E., Besser, G.M. and Rees, L.H. (1986) 'Cushing's Syndrome', *Clinics in Endocrinology and Metabolism, 14,* in Press

Jeffcoate, W.J. and Edwards, C.R.W. (1979) 'Cushing's Syndrome; Pathogenesis, Diagnosis and Treatment', in V.H.T. James (ed.), *The Adrenal Gland,* pp. 165-98, Raven Press, New York

Krieger, D.T. (1983) 'Physiopathology of Cushing's Disease', *Endocrine Reviews, 4,* 22-43

12 THE POSTERIOR PITUITARY

Historical Introduction

Although only a small gland, the posterior pituitary has an important place in endocrine history. The active principles of the posterior pituitary were extracted relatively early — around the turn of the century — and their activities identified. Following the description in 1895 by Oliver and Schäfer of a vasopressor substance in the mammalian pituitary, it was accepted that the prime function of the neurohypophysis was the regulation of blood pressure. A few years later, in 1906, Dale described its 'oxytocic' activity — the ability to produce uterine contractions. Blair Bell in 1909 injected posterior pituitary extracts into pregnant women, and thus introduced the use of such extracts into clinical obstetric practice. The doses used tended to be very high, and in 1927 Bourne and Burn stressed the efficacy of much smaller doses. In 1948, Theobald showed that an infusion of 2.5 mU/min oxytocin (Pituitrin standardised for oxytocin) was sufficient to stimulate uterine contractions. An action on the mammary gland was recognised in 1910 by Ott and Scott, who noted that extracts of the posterior pituitary stimulated milk flow, an observation confirmed in 1911 by Schäfer and Mackenzie. Gaines was the first to distinguish clearly the process of milk ejection from that of secretion, and he presented the first evidence that injection of pituitary extracts stimulated natural milk ejection. It was originally believed that the neural lobe promoted diuresis, but in 1913 Farini and Van den Velden independently demonstrated an antidiuretic action of extracts of the neural lobe in patients with diabetes insipidus, the daily urine volumes being in the region of 6 litres. Subsequently, in 1924, Starling and Verney reported that the neural lobe acted directly on the kidney to produce its effects. The use of the toad bladder *in vitro* as a model for studying the action of antidiuretic hormone was foreshadowed by the studies in 1921 of Brunner, who showed that the permeability of frog skin to water was increased by neurohypophysial principles. However, although the four major activities of the neurohypophysial principles (oxytocic, milk-ejecting, pressor and antidiuretic) were discovered early in this century, the subsequent development of knowledge of the neurohypophysis was slow. This is possibly because the conditions associated with excess or deficiency of the hormones are rare; and it is such clinical observations which have led — and still do lead — to a greater understanding of the role of any hormone. There has been no syndrome described that is associated with over- or underproduction of oxytocin. For many years, the only condition associated with disturbance of neurohypophysial function was diabetes insipidus, a condition in which the patient produces copious amounts of dilute urine as a result of partial or complete lack of vasopressin. It was not until 1957 that the syndrome associated with overproduction of vasopressin was described: the Schwartz-Barrter syndrome or SIADH.

154   *The Posterior Pituitary*

Structure

Oxytocin was the first hormone to be isolated and purified, to have its amino acid sequence established and finally to be synthesised. This was carried out independently by two groups of workers, one in the laboratories of Du Vigneaud and the other in those of Acher. This was a considerable scientific feat, for although nowadays a new analogue or antagonist may be synthesised in as little as three weeks, at that time it was a very lengthy procedure. Oxytocin and vasopressin were found to comprise nine amino acids and to have molecular weights around 1000 (Figure 12.1). The two hormones are virtually identical, differing merely

Figure 12.1: Structure of Oxytocin and Vasopressin

Arginine Vasopressin

$$\begin{array}{ccc} 3 & 2 & 1 \\ \text{Phe} - \text{Tyr} - \text{Cys} \\ | & & | \\ \text{Gln} - \text{Asn} - \text{Cys} - \text{Pro} - \text{Arg} - \text{Gly (NH}_2) \\ 4 & 5 & 6 & 7 & 8 & 9 \end{array}$$

Oxytocin

$$\begin{array}{ccc} 3 & 2 & 1 \\ \text{Ile} - \text{Ty} - \text{Cys} \\ | & & | \\ \text{Gln} - \text{Asn} - \text{Cys} - \text{Pro} - \text{Leu} - \text{Gly (NH}_2) \\ 4 & 5 & 6 & 7 & 8 & 9 \end{array}$$

in the residues in postions 3 and 8. There is a disulphide bridge between the cystine residues in positions 1 and 6, so that the hormone is 'tadpole-like', with a head or ring portion and a tail portion. Whereas the amino acid composition of most peptide hormones varies from species to species, oxytocin and vasopressin are the same throughout the entire mannalian kingdom, with the exception of the 'suiforms', i.e. the pig, the peccary and the hippopotamus, in which lysine vasopressin occurs as opposed to arginine vasopressin. This is of some interest as lysine vasopressin has been used to treat diabetes insipidus in man. When discussing the hormones, one should strictly speak of lysine vasopressin or arginine vasopressin, but generally the term vasopressin alone is used, usually referring to the latter. Initially, when the active principle was isolated it was called vasopressin because of its effect on blood pressure. When the antidiuretic activity was found to be the most important property of the hormone, it became 'antidiuretic hormone'. Now that the composition of the hormone is known, it has been given the chemical name 'arginine vasopressin'. Once the structure of oxytocin and vasopressin had been demonstrated, many analogues of the hormones were synthesised, largely with a view to identifying which residues were important for action. In several instances, analogues were synthesised that were subsequently shown to occur in non-mammalian species. With modifications chiefly in positions 3, 4 and 8, neuro-hypophysial hormones are found throughout the vertebrate species, bearing such exotic names as glumitocin and vasotocin, the latter being a putative pineal neurohormone.

Neurosecretory Neurones

In addition to the fact that the hormones of the neurohypophysial system were the first to be synthesised, this system was the first to provide evidence of neurosecretion. Although it is now well established that neurones may produce a whole variety of peptide products, at the time the concept that neurones could produce hormones in addition to classical neurotransmitters was a very exciting one, one that allowed true integration of the nervous and endocrine control systems. This concept was largley due to the work of Bargmann and Scharrer, who perfected a histological technique which stained neurosecretory products. Using this technique, they were able to demonstrate a pathway passing from the hypothalamus to the posterior pituitary. They also showed that, following stalk section (with a barrier placed across the site of section), material accumulated in the axons proximal to the block whereas the axons distal to this point were relatively free of neurosecretory staining material. This demonstrated that the hormones or precursors were synthesised in the hypothalamus and transported along the hypothalamo-hypophysial tract to the posterior pituitary. Oxytocin and vasopressin are synthesised in the perikarya of the supraoptic and paraventricular nuclei, i.e. the magnocellular nuclei, so-called because of the relatively large size of the cells. They are typical actively-secreting cells, with abundant rough endoplasmic reticulum, well-developed Golgi bodies and neurosecretory granules 150–200 nm in diameter. The terminals also contain smaller granules 50–60 nm in diameter, which may arise through rupture of the membranes following secretion. There are some non-secreting terminals in the posterior pituitary containing only small vesicles. Pituicytes, probably a type of glial cell, are also found in the posterior pituitary. Their function is unclear, but they may be involved in information processing as peptide receptors have been demonstrated on their surfaces. Oxytocin and vasopressin are synthesised in separate neurones found in both the paraventricular and supraoptic nuclei. Immunocytochemical techniques have also revealed a greater number of vasopressin-containing cells in the supraoptic nucleus.

The two hormones are associated in the neurohypophysis with their so-called carrier proteins, the neurophysins. The neurophysins were first described a little over twenty years ago, and are a family of proteins with a molecular weight of 9000–10 000, i.e. some ten times that of the hormone. It appears that in most species there are two major neurophysins. These have been termed neurophysin I and neurophysin II, although other forms of nomenclature have been put forward, depending, for example, on the terminal amino acid sequence. The partial or complete amino acid sequence has been determined for neurophysins from a number of species, and the structure appears to be relatively conserved. Within the neurosecretory neurones, vasopressin is associated with neurophysin I, and oxytocin with neurophysin II. No systemic role for the neurophysins has been described; although they do not appear to bind the hormones in the circulation,

156 *The Posterior Pituitary*

they may do so in the pituitary. However, it is possible that they merely represent by-products of synthesis, and are without other functions.

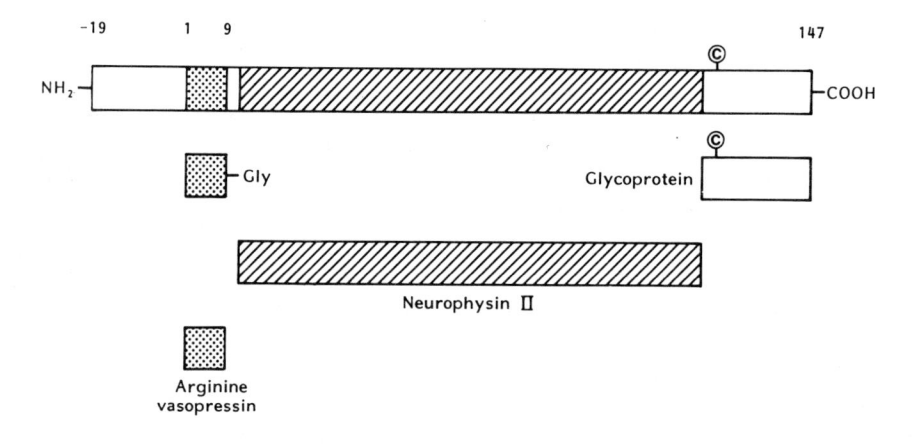

Synthesis and Secretion

Understanding of the mechanisms of synthesis of neurohypophysial hormones, particularly vasopressin, stemmed from the work of Sachs and his co-workers. The hormone is synthesised, together with its accompanying peptide, neurophysin, in the form of a precursor molecule. The oxytocin and vasopressin pre-prohormones have been sequenced. The vasopressin precursor contains 116 amino acids, of which 19 appear to belong to the 'signal' sequence (Figure 12.2). This signal sequence, which begins with Met-14 at the N-terminus, is immediately followed by the arginine vasopressin sequence, which is in turn separated from the neurophysin II sequence by Gly-Lys-Arg. This in turn is separated from the 39 C-terminal glycopeptide moiety by a single Arg. The oxytocin precursor molecule also contains oxytocin and oxytocin-associated neurophysin, but has no terminal glycoprotein residue. Once synthesised, the complex is packaged within the neurosecretory granules and transported to the posterior lobe (Figure 12.3). Studies using bioassay techniques reveal that the active hormone is formed during this process of transport. Transport occurs at the rate of 2–3 mm/h, some ten times greater than the normally observed axoplasmic flow, so some special transport mechanism must be involved, probably employing microtubules. As

Figure 12.2: Diagram Showing the Structure of the Vasopressin Precursor Molecule and its Subsequent Cleavage to AVP and Neurophysin II

Figure 12.3: Synthesis and Secretion of Vasopressin

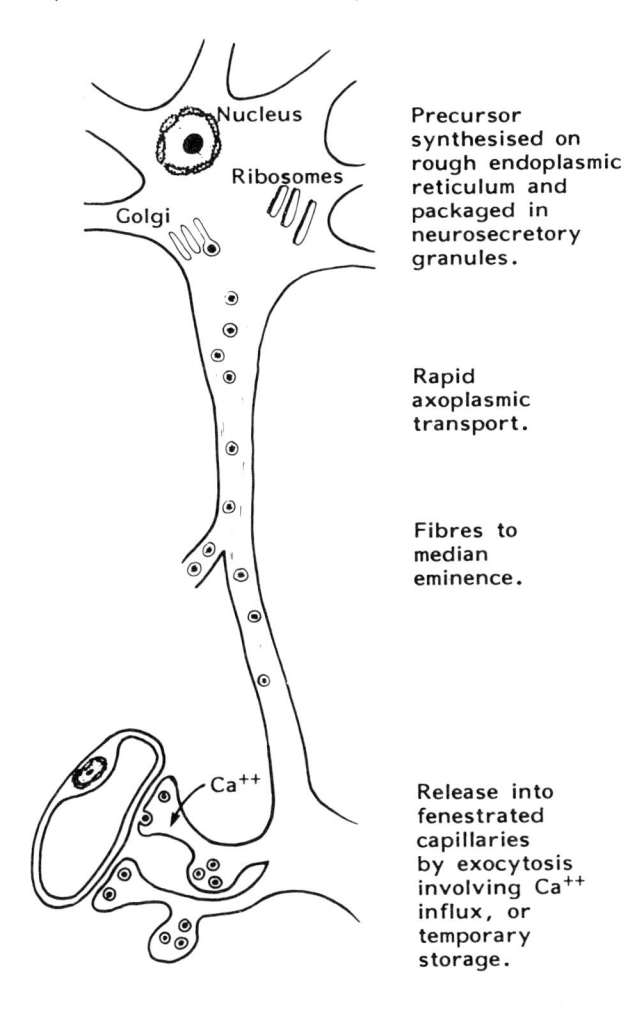

Precursor synthesised on rough endoplasmic reticulum and packaged in neurosecretory granules.

Rapid axoplasmic transport.

Fibres to median eminence.

Release into fenestrated capillaries by exocytosis involving Ca^{++} influx, or temporary storage.

with other neurotransmitters/neuromodulators, the most recently synthesised molecules are the first to be released. Material newly-arrived in the nerve terminal congregates at neurosecretory sites in preparation for release into the adjacent fenestrated capillaries. That which is not released moves into nerve terminals for storage. Recently it has been shown that vasopressin-containing pathways pass not only to the posterior piuitary but also to the median eminence. Any vasopressin released at this site might influence the release of ACTH. Extra-hypothalamic pathways containing vasopressin and oxytocin have also been found, and have been suggested to play a role in memory processes.

Nerve action potentials travelling down the hypothalamo-hypophysial tract cause the release of hormone from the nerve terminals by exocytosis. Both excitatory and inhibitory influences act upon the supraoptic and paraventricular nuclei. Only two pathways have been established, which project directly to the supraoptic nucleus, a large noradrenergic projection arising from the A1 neurones in the ventrolateral medulla, and a projection from the subfornical organ. Other regions of the central nervous system have been shown to alter the activity of the supraoptic nucleus, but probably do not project directly to this region. In addition to the adrenergic inputs, other afferent connections have been proposed, including cholinergic, histaminergic, GABAergic, serotoninergic and opioid. The paraventricular nucleus is considerably more complex than the supraoptic nucleus containing both parvicellular and magnocellular divisions. The magnocellular division in turn can be further subdivided on the basis of efferent projections to areas of the central nervous system other than the neural lobe. Functionally, the paraventricular nucleus is again more complicated than the supraoptic. In addition to regulating the function of the neurohypophysis, it appears to participate in the regulation of food intake, ACTH release from the anterior pituitary, and possibly modulation of cardiovascular reflexes. The afferents to the supraoptic nucleus are similarly represented in the paraventricular nucleus.

The rate of release of vasopressin has been correlated with the pattern of firing of antidromically-identified magnocellular neurones in the rat. Putative vasopressin neurones may be distinguished from putative oxytocin neurones according to their behaviour during reflex milk ejection. At this time the oxytocin cells show a high-frequency discharge pattern, whereas vasopressin neurones are not activated. There are three basic types of firing pattern that have been described in the supraoptic and paraventricular nuclei: slow irregular, continuous and phasic firing. Under certain conditions a phasic pattern of action potentials is seen during stimulation of vasopressin release. Dehydration of rats causes a change from slow irregular to a phasic pattern. It appears that this is the most efficient way of stimulating hormone release from these neurones. Patterns of firing of oxytocin neurones have also been characterised in the rat. Typically, rat pups attach themselves to the mother's nipples for 18 h out of the 24. Milk ejection occurs every 4–8 min, and about 18 s before the rise in intramammary pressure there is a burst of firing.

The linking of electrical events to hormone release is called stimulus-secretion coupling and is dependent upon calcium ions. The presence of these ions results in fusion of the membranes of the neurosecretory granules with the cell membranes, and both hormone and neurophysin are released by exocytosis into capillaries on to which the nerve endings abut. The membrane of each of the neurosecretory granules is taken back into the cell and is believed to form vacuoles, as already mentioned. Oxytocin and vasopressin are generally released separately.

Vasopressin

Control of Vasopressin Release

Vasopressin is readily released in response to a number of stimuli. The principal physiological stimulus for release is an increase in the osmotic pressure of the extracellular fluid. This was elegantly demonstrated by Verney in 1947 in a series of experiments in conscious dogs. He infused sufficient hypertonic saline into one carotid artery to increase the tonicity of the blood passing to the head by 2 per cent and was able to demonstrate as a result the inhibition of a water diuresis. By successively ligating the blood vessels in the region, he subsequently located the areas sensitive to osmotic stimuli in the anterior hypothalamus. Although these studies were performed over thirty years ago, the manner in which the osmotic change is monitored is not known; indeed, even the cells involved have not been identified. Some workers believe that the magnocellular cells themselves are sensitive to changes in osmotic pressure, whereas others believe that the receptors are independent of magnocellular neurones. More recently, as a result of studies on the conscious goat in which a number of osmotically-active substances were injected directly into the cerebral ventricles, Anderson has challenged the view of osmoreceptors and has suggested that one should think in terms of sodium receptors. Whatever the underlying mechanism, it has been shown by making accurate determinations of vasopressin and plasma osmolality that there is a close relationship between the two. Under normal conditions when the plasma osmolality lies in the region of 290 mOsm/kg, the plasma vasopressin concentration is the order of 1 μU/ml (2.2 pmol/litre).

This close relationship between vasopressin and osmolality is influenced by the circulating plasma volume. The volume of the extracellular fluid is just one of a number of non-osmotic influences on vasopressin release. Some of these factors are listed in Table 12.1. It can be seen that vasopressin is readily released in response to a number of stimuli. Volume changes provide a very potent stimulus whereas osmoreceptors are the most sensitive. Vasopressin release is stimulated by a rise in osmolality of 1 per cent, whereas a 10 per cent fall in blood volume is required to increase hormone secretion. Volume-induced release is thought to occur through receptors in the atria and great veins sensitive to low pressure. About 70 per cent of the circulating blood is in the low-pressure system, so that receptors in this area are sensitive to the degree of vascular filling. High-pressure receptors or baroreceptors, situated in the carotid and aortic arch, also act in response to types of blood loss sufficient to produce a fall in blood pressure. The afferent pathways for these responses lie in the vagus, glossopharyngeal and aortic nerves. Evidence for the role of baroreceptors comes from experiments involving the study of haemorrhage and carotid occlusion, with vagus and sinus nerves cut or left intact. Similarly, experiments with afferent nerves sectioned before stimulation of the atrial receptors have been used to demonstrate their importance. It appears that the diuresis seen upon atrial distension is due in part to reduced vasopressin secretion and in part to the release of a natriuretic peptide, possibly the recently identified atrial natriuretic peptide.

In situations in which water retention is important, such as at high temperatures, one might expect increased vasopressin release; indeed the experimental results support this hypothesis. Another environmental change that results in enhanced vasopressin secretion is a fall in pO_2 as seen at altitude. Retention of CO_2 may have a similar effect. The physiological relevance of these remains uncertain.

As with many anterior pituitary hormones, stresses such as the pain and trauma

160 The Posterior Pituitary

Table 12.1: Non-osmotic Factors Postulated to Influence Vasopressin Release

Pain and irritation
Emotion and anxiety
Conditioned reflexes
Surgery
Exercise
Environmental 'stress'
Changes in environmental temperature

Expansion and contraction of blood volume
Contraction and expansion of extracellular fluid volume
Distribution of blood
Changes in blood pressure
Changes in blood gas tensions

Hormones including:
    Angiotensin
    Catecholamines
    Steroids   cortisol
                   oestrogen
                   progesterone
                   testosterone
Drugs including:
    Opiates
    Alcohol
    Nicotine
    Carbamazepine
    Thioridazine
    Clofibrate

associated with surgery can also stimulate vasopressin release (Figure 12.4). As well as the central nervous stimuli, which can affect vasopressin release in the absence of changes in plasma osmolality or blood pressure, a number of hormones have been said to stimulate vasopressin release. It has been claimed that angiotensin II, catecholamines and certain steroids all have this effect, but it is not clear if all these observations are physiologically important. For example, circulating angiotensin II is only effective in concentrations not seen under physiological conditions. Changes in the plasma concentrations of steroid hormones may, however, be of importance in regulating the release of neurohypophysial hormones. Concentrations of oxytocin and vasopressin in plasma vary over the menstrual cycle, being highest at the time of ovulation and lowest at the onset of menstruation. This pattern of vasopressin secretion can also be reproduced by administering oestrogen and progesterone to post-menopausal women, oestradiol appearing to stimulate and progesterone to inhibit hormone release. Probably the best-known substance recognised as influencing vasopressin release is alcohol, and there is no need to cite the evidence confirming this. Anaesthetics in general were at one time thought to stimulate vasopressin release directly, but it is now thought that the effect is secondary to accompanying changes such as a fall in blood pressure.

Release of vasopressin in response to an increase in plasma osmolality and a fall in circulating blood volume is part of a series of homeostatic mechanisms

Figure 12.4: Release of Vasopressin (Vertical Axis) during Coronary Bypass Surgery. Blood samples taken at anaesthetic induction (PI) and intubation (INT), and at 3-min intervals at leg incision (LEG), sternotomy (CHEST, SAW, SPREADER), pericardial traction (PERI) and at various times on bypass (CPB)

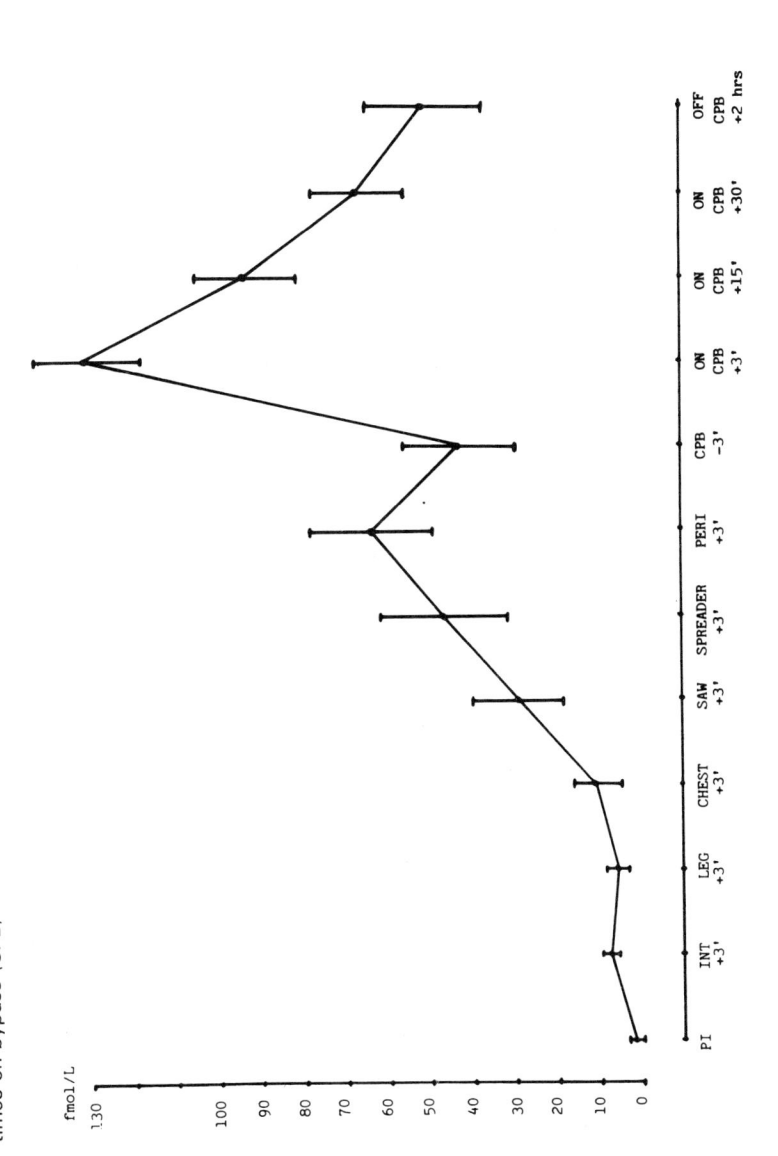

162 The Posterior Pituitary

Figure 12.5: Role of Vasopressin in Maintaining Extracellular Fluid Volume

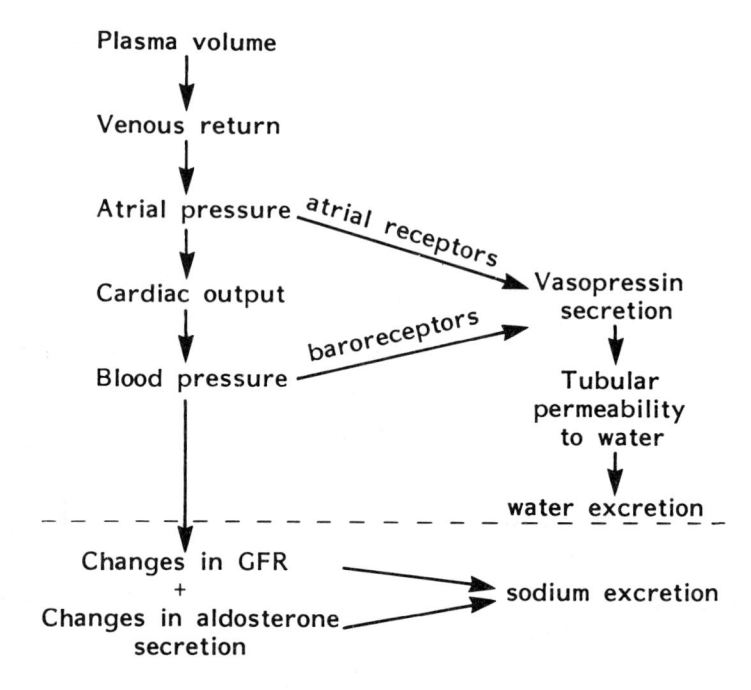

```
Plasma volume
      ↓
Venous return
      ↓
Atrial pressure ──atrial receptors──┐
      ↓                              ↓
Cardiac output              Vasopressin
      ↓          baroreceptors  secretion
Blood pressure ─────────────→       ↓
      │                        Tubular
      │                        permeability
      │                        to water
      │                              ↓
 ─ ─ ─┼─ ─ ─ ─ ─ ─ ─ ─ ─ ─ ─ ─ water excretion ─ ─
      ↓
Changes in GFR ────────────┐
      +                     → sodium excretion
Changes in aldosterone ────┘
      secretion
```

regulating extracellular fluid volume, in particular that of the circulating blood volume (Figure 12.5). It is not so obvious what the role of vasopressin following stress could be, although it is tempting to speculate that it is linked to two recently described vasopressin actions, namely an effect on learning in rats and an ability to stimulate glycogenolysis.

Metabolism

Once released into the circulation, vasopressin is rapidly cleared, with a half-time a little over five minutes. The principal site of clearance is the kidney, although the liver probably contributes to the process. Vasopressin appears to circulate in the unbound form, there being no significant association with neurophysin or any other protein once it is secreted into the circulation.

Action of Vasopressin

Of the 150 litres of fluid filtered daily, about 85 per cent is reabsorbed in the proximal convoluted tubule. Reabsorption of the remaining fluid is largely under the control of vasopressin. Normally 1.5 litres of urine per day are excreted, with an osmolality in the range of 400–800 mOsm/kg. In the absence of vasopressin, this is increased to 20 litres per day and the osmolality is reduced to 30–60 mOsm/kg. The same amount of solute is excreted, the fall in concentration resulting from the additional volume of water excreted. Vasopressin thus acts on reabsorption of water. If the urine is more dilute than plasma, then it may be assumed that circulating vasopressin concentrations are minimal or absent. Studies on the isolated collecting duct have shown that vasopressin increases the permeability of this duct to water. This allows water to flow out of the collecting duct, down the osmotic gradient produced by the counter-current mechanism of the loop of Henle. Much of our knowledge of the way in which vasopressin brings about permeability changes in the mammalian renal tubule has come from studies on amphibian membranes, in particular the toad bladder. This preparation appears to respond to vasopressin in a similar way to the renal tubule. Vassopressin acts on the tubule cells from the basal (blood) side but exerts its effect on the apical (urinary) side. Water absorbed from the tubule leaves partly via the lateral cell membranes and enters the lateral intracellular space. As with other peptide hormones, cyclic AMP seems to be the mediator of the vasopressin response (Figure 12.6). Vasopressin receptors on the basal side of the collecting duct membranes are functionally linked to adenylate cyclase. The rise in cyclic AMP produced by stimulation of this enzyme leads to protein kinase activation and the phosphorylation of one or more protein substrates at the luminal membrane of the epithelial cells. This phosphorylation has been postulated to be involved in the changes in luminal water permeability, but no direct experimental evidence to support this postulate has been provided. There is, however, considerable evidence from electron-microscopic studies to indicate the reorganisation in the structure of the luminal membrane accompanying the change in water permeability. A membrane 'shuttle' hypothesis has been formulated to explain the action of vasopressin on apical or luminal membrane water permeability. On exposure to the hormone, portions of the membrane highly permeable to water are shuttled from cytoplasmic vacuoles to the luminal plasma membrane with which they then fuse. This fusion results in marked increases in the water permeability of the membrane. The water-retaining action of vasopressin is produced by low concentrations of the hormone. Maximum urine concentration is produced by a vasopresssin concentration of 5 μu/ml.

At concentrations higher than those required to produce an antidiuresis, vasopressin can act on the cardiovascular system producing vasoconstriction and an increase in blood pressure. It may also have a direct effect on the heart, producing bradycardia. Some vascular beds, as, for example, that of the splanchnic region, are more sensitive to vasopressin than others. This is of importance in the use of vasopressin infusion to prevent bleeding from the gastro-intestinal tract. It was thought that as relatively high doses vasopressin are required to produce a change in blood pressure, this action of the hormone was not of physiological significance. However, more recent studies have suggested that vasopressin may play a part in the regulation of blood pressure and in the aetiology of hypertension, although the current status of vasopressin in blood-pressure regulation remains controversial.

It is likely that vasopressin released into the portal blood from the median eminence plays a role in ACTH release and is part of the CRF-macromolecular complex. Several other actions have been described for vasopressin, but are only seen in the presence of relatively high concentrations of vasopressin. These actions

Figure 12.6: Postulated Mechanism of Vasopressin Action on the Renal Tubule Cell. AC, adenylate cyclase; TJ, tight junction; MF, microfilament; I, cytoplasmic tubule with water conduction particles; II, delivery of particles to luminal membrane following fusion; III, particles aggregated on luminal membrane

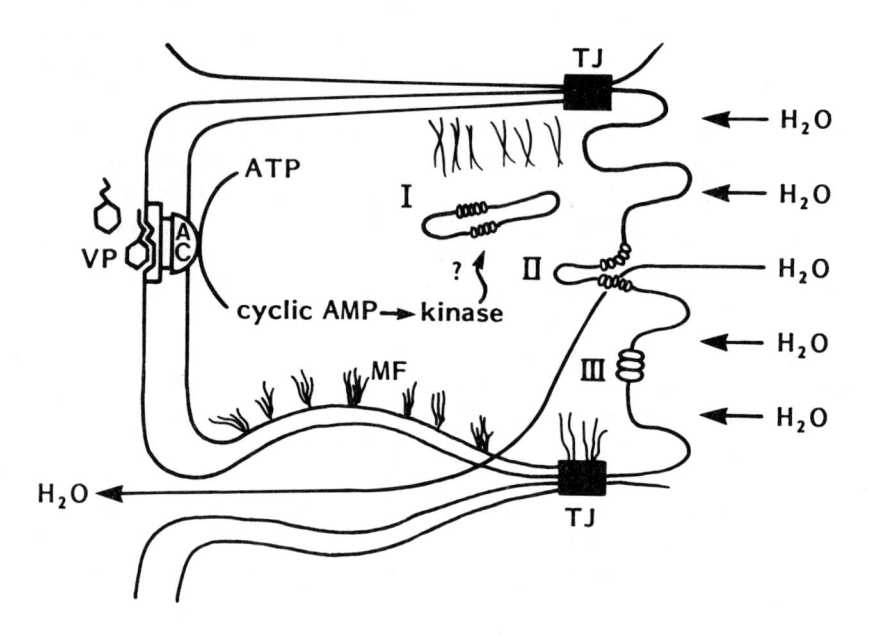

include stimulation of hepatic glycogenolysis, an action on fibrinolysis and all components of the factor VIII system, and potentiation of the acquisition of conditioned reflexes. The fact that experiments in rats suggested that vasopressin facilitates memory consolidation and retrieval whereas oxytocin appeared to be amnesic has excited considerable interest. That the central nervous effects of these hormones is indeed of central origin has been indicated in a number of ways, including lesion studies and administration of peptides and specific antisera in particular brain areas. Neurochemical experiments have suggested that the effects of neurohypophysial hormones are modulation of catecholamine transmission in restricted areas of the brain. The effects of neurohypophysial hormones on memory processes and other central nervous effects are dissociated from their classical endocrine function and are probably caused by neuropeptides generated from these hormones. Structure-activity and biotransformation studies corroborate the hypothesis that vasopressin and oxytocin are precursor molecules of the second order of neuropeptides with specific effects on memory processes. It must be confessed that some workers remain sceptical as to the significance of behavioural studies in rats. The clinical trials with vasopressin-like peptides are even more difficult to evaluate, as there are many sources of difference and error. However, it is claimed that these peptides have behavioural effects in humans and may be of potential value in affective illness.

Oxytocin

Relatively fewer studies have been performed on the release and action of oxytocin than on vasopressin. It appears that although oxytocin is present in the pituitaries of both male and female experimental animals in similar amounts to that of vasopressin, it has no clear role in the male, although it may be released during mating and appears to be released in the female largely during parturition and lactation and possibly during mating. The release, like that of vasopressin, may be regarded as the efferent limb of a neuroendocrine reflex. The receptors lie in the region of the nipple and cervix. Thus, stretching of the lower genital tract leads to oxytocin release and subsequent milk let-down, a response known as Ferguson's reflex. This reflex was first described in 1942, although herdsmen had been aware of it for centuries and had used it during milking. In the second century AD, Galen described how herdsmen would blow down horn pipes into the vaginas of mares to improve milk yield.

As with other hypothalamic hormones, oxytocin is secreted in an episodic fashion. Oxytocin release is affected by higher centres so that stress under certain circumstances can suppress oxytocin release. Thus, nursing mothers are sometimes unable to breast feed successfully if stressed or upset. Although stimulation of the nipple contributes to oxytocin release during suckling, other factors may be involved, such as the sight and the sound of the infant. The relative concentrations of oxytocin found in the plasma are higher during parturition than lactation, the concentrations being low initially and increasing as labour progresses. The highest concentrations have been reported with the expulsion of the fetus. However, it should be noted that early studies purporting to show an increase in circulating oxytocin during pregnancy may have been confounded by the increase in plasma oxytocinase. This enzyme degrades oxytocin, and can thus decrease the activity of radio-labelled oxytocin. In an RIA, this fall in radio-labelled oxytocin bound to antibody may be falsely ascribed to increasing levels of oxytocin in the plasma sample. Oxytocin does not therefore seem to be important in the initiation of parturition, but is important in the expulsion of the placenta and fetus. In recent studies oxytocin has been detected in cord blood during delivery and in the blood of chronically-catheterised sheep fetuses in the 48 hours before parturition, which raises the exciting possibility that in some species fetal oxytocin may play a role in parturition. Certainly oxytocin infusion into the sheep fetus can produce uterine contractions. There is also recent evidence that the ovary is a source of oxytocin; this may relate to the onset of menstruation (see below).

Actions of Oxytocin

Oxytocin acts on the uterus to produce an increase in the number and strength of contractions. It may also influence the production of prostaglandins, which will in turn stimulate uterine contraction. The sensitivity of the uterus to the hormone depends on the steroid background, progesterone being inhibitory and oestrogens facilitatory. At the time of parturition, maternal progesterone concentrations fall and oestrogen concentrations increase, so that the uterine sensitivity is modified and will respond to oxytocin concentrations which were ineffective at earlier stages of pregnancy. This increased sensitivity is due to the induction of oxytocin receptors by oestrogen. The action of oxytocin on the uterus is employed clinically to induce labour. Changes in the uterine sensitivity at full term must, of course, be considered when oxytocin is used to this end. Although widely used, oxytocin infusions may produce some adverse effects, the chief of which appears to be fetal hyperbilirubinaemia. This may be a consequence of the relative immaturity of the fetus rather than a direct action of oxytocin. It has also been recently suggested that the increased oxytocin release during sexual intercourse may facilitate the movement of sperm into the Fallopian tube.

Relatively less research has been carried out on the mechanism of contraction of smooth muscle as compared with skeletal muscle. Consequently, the underlying mechanisms are less well understood. It is thought that oxytocin acts on the myometrial cells to alter the resting potential so that the cells depolarise more readily. Again, the exact nature of the oxytocin action on the mammary gland is not clearly established, but it appears to cause contraction of the myoepithelial cells. These cells encircle the alveoli and ducts of the mammary gland, such that when they contract the alveoli reduce in size and the ducts become wider. Milk is thus expressed from the alveoli and into the main ducts. The action of oxytocin does not seem to be accompanied by an increase in cyclic AMP. There is little evidence as to the molecular changes responsible for the effects, but it has been suggested that an increase in cyclic GMP may cause contraction whereas an increase in cyclic AMP may cause relaxation.

Oxytocin may have yet another function associated with reproduction, namely, in regression of the corpus luteum. Some time ago oxytocin was shown to be luteolytic in the cow and the goat, and the presence of oxytocin in the ovary has awakened interest in this observation. It is proposed that the effect is caused indirectly by stimulating release of prostaglandin from the uterine endometrium, although recent evidence has suggested that oxytocin can directly inhibit steroidogenesis. The mechanism of luteolysis in the human is not well characterised, but a possible role for oxytocin is of obvious interest as this may be relevant to formulating non-steroidal contraceptive agents.

Investigators are still looking for a role for oxytocin in the male, apart from the possible effect on sperm transport. The most likely possibility appears to be an action on salt excretion. Oxytocin in supra-physiological concentrations has been demonstrated to enhance sodium chloride excretion in a number of species, but recently it has also been shown in the hypophysectomised rat that oxytocin and vasopressin act synergistically in this respect, so that salt excretion is promoted with very low levels of oxytocin infusion. However, whether this is relevant to man remains speculative.

Disorders of Neurohypophysial Function

Clinically significant diseases of the posterior pituitary are uncommon. From the endocrine standpoint they can be divided into conditions caused by increased or decreased vasopressin secretion. There are no known conditions, obstetric or otherwise, resulting from a deficiency or excess of oxytocin secretion. Women with posterior pituitary dysfunction resulting in diabetes insipidus have normal pregnancies and deliveries. Space-occupying lesions sufficient to cause disturbances of vasopressin release usually also causes local symptoms such as headache and visual disturbances. They may also lead to changes in adenohypophysial activity.

Neurohypophysial function may be disturbed with lesions in the hypothalamo-hypophysial stalk or neural lobe. The classification of the pathological changes in the neurohypophysis can be based on morphological changes. Interruption of the stalk by surgical sections or trauma results in the atrophy of supraoptic and paraventricular nuclei as well as of the posterior lobe. Basophil invasion is a common histological finding, but cannot be correlated with any endocrine abnormality. Squamous cell nests, glandular structures and focal lymphocyte infiltration are also common findings in the posterior lobe or pituitary stalk. Various granulomas — tuberculosis, sarcoidosis and syphilis — may be present in the stalk and neural lobe. External destruction may lead to diabetes insipidus. Similarly, haemorrhage and necrosis, although uncommon, may lead to diabetes insipidus. These may be associated with traumatic head injuries, post-partum necrosis of the anterior pituitary, increased intracranial pressure, shock, or haematological disorders leading to a tendency to bleed. Neoplasms of the posterior pituitary are uncommon; from the endocrine viewpoint metastatic carcinomas are the most important. Neurohypophysial metastases are not rare, but occur more frequently than in the adenohypophysis. Granular cell tumours are the most commonly occurring primary neurohypophysial tumours. Generally such tumours are symptomless, but occasionally may lead to diabetes insipidus. Neoplasms of the infundibulum are very rare. These may occasionally invade the pituitary stalk, neural lobe or optic nerve, and may extend to involve the mamillary bodies, hypothalamus or third ventricle, and, by compression, displacement or destruction of these regions may produce endocrine abnormalities.

Inappropriate Secretion of Vasopressin

In 1957 Schwartz, Bennet, Curelop and Barrter described two patients with carcinoma of the bronchus who, despite hyponatraemia, continued to excrete a concentrated urine. The syndrome was similar to the response of normal subjects given an infusion of Pitressin and water, and it was therefore postulated that the tumour was associated with inappropriate secretion of vasopressin. The cardinal features of this syndrome (Table 12.2), usually termed the syndrome of inappropriate antidiuretic hormone secretion (SIADH), are hyponatraemia with hypo-osmolality of the plasma and extracellulare fluid, continued renal excretion of sodium with inappropriately high urine osmolality, the absence of clinical evidence of volume depletion or oedema, and normal renal and adrenal function. The consequences of the chronic hyponatraemia are thirst, impaired taste and anorexia, accompanied by dyspnoea on exercise and fatigue when the plasma sodium falls from normal to 130 mmol/litre. Nausea, vomiting and abdominal cramps occur if there is a further fall to 120 mmol/litre. Below 115 mmol/litre, confusion, lethargy, muscle twitching, convulsions and death may occur. Patients with SIADH usually retain 2–5 litres of excess water and remain in a new steady state with a low serum sodium.

Table 12.2: Laboratory Findings in the Syndrome of Inappropriate Vasopressin Secretion

	Total body content	Intracellular content	Plasma content	Urine content
Free water	Increased	—	Increased	Reduced
Osmolality	—	—	Reduced	Increased
Sodium	Normal	Increased	Reduced	Increased
Potassium	Reduced	Reduced	Reduced	Increased

The original report of SIADH was in association with bronchogenic carcinoma, and since then the syndrome has been described in association with many tumours. It now appears that ectopic hormone production by tumours is quite common, although the clinical manifestation of the associated syndrome is rare. Inappropriate vasopressin secretion is also seen in patients with diseases of the central nervous system such as bacterial meningitis, cerebral tuberculosis, subarachnoid bleeding, psychiatric disease and head injury or respiratory disease including bronchopneumonia and tuberculosis (Table 12.3). It is also seen in association with a number of other diseases, those in which it is most frequently reported being myxoedema and acute intermittent porphyria. Hyponatraemia with a clinical profile identical to that seen in SIADH has been described after treatment with various drugs such as clofibrate, carbamazepine, antineoplastic agents such as vinblastine, and neuroleptics. Chlorpropamide may cause hyponatraemia by sensitising the renal tubule to vasopressin rather than by directly increasing its secretion.

Table 12.3: Conditions Associated with the Syndrome of Inappropriate Vasopressin Secretion

Tumours,	e.g.	bronchogenic, oesophageal and bladder carcinomas
Central nervous system disease,	e.g.	bacterial meningitis, cerebral tuberculosis, subarachnoid haemorrhage, cerebral thrombosis, head injury, psychiatric disease, dementia
Respiratory disease,	e.g.	tuberculosis, bronchopneumonia, empyema
Other diseases	e.g.	myxodema, cirrhosis, acute intermittent porphyria
Drugs,	e.g.	vinblastine, clofibrate, carbamazepine

The choice of treatment depends on the severity of the hyponatraemia, the rapidity with which it developed, and the severity of the clinical symptoms. When the serum sodium falls below 100 mmol/litre, or when neurological symptoms are observed, rapid correction of the hyponatraemia with hypertonic saline should be attempted. Restitution of the blood osmolality can also be accomplished by giving frusemide (plus salt supplements) which results in the production of urine approximately isotonic to plasma. In relatively asymptomatic patients and those in which the plasma sodium is above 115 mmol/litre, treatment may be accomplished by restricting water to 800 ml per day while continuing to provide excess dietary sodium. In the long term, the only satisfactory treatment is the relief of the cause, which may be relatively straightforward when it involves discontinuation of a drug, treatment of a pulmonary infection, or replacement of an endocrine deficiency. In difficult cases, demethylchlortetracycline can be used to render the renal tubule refractory to vasopressin, although it is likely to cause photosensitivity. Lithium salts are more toxic and less effective (nephrogenic diabetes insipidus as seen in 30 per cent of patients on lithium medication).

Diabetes Insipidus

Diabetes insipidus is due to vasopressin deficiency and is characterised by polyuria and polydipsia. It may develop in patients with organic lesions of the hypothalamus, pituitary stalk or neural lobe. Morphologically diverse lesions are evident in the hypothalamus, especially in the supraoptic nucleus. Destruction of the posterior lobe results in only slight or moderate temporary polyuria and polydipsia, as the site of synthesis of vasopressin is not destroyed. Organic lesions include various tumours, metastatic carcinomas, granulomas, traumatic injuries, histiocytosis X, meningo-encephalitis, lymphomas and leukaemias. Around 30 percent of cases of diabetes insipidus are idiopathic; in these no gross destructive lesion can be demonstrated in the hypothalamus, stalk or pituitary lobe, although careful histological studies may reveal various organic abnormalities such as a reduction in the size and number of cells in the magnocellular nuclei. Such patients also have a high incidence of vasopressin neurone antibodies, suggesting that this may be part of the spectrum of autoimmune disease. A high incidence of such antibodies is also seen in patients with histiocytosis X.

Idiopathic diabetes insipidus represents the largest group with deficiency of vasopressin. Some cases are familial, usually autosomal dominant or recessive. Brain tumours and head trauma are the next most frequently reported causes. The diagnosis of diabetes insipidus is based on evaluation of the hypothalamo-hypophysial system, and is most conveniently carried out using a dehydration test in which fluids are withheld for a given period of time (Chapter 14). Care should be taken to avoid severe dehydration by not allowing the body weight to fall by more than 5 per cent. At the end of dehydration, vasopressin may be administered and the renal response observed. If the neurohypophysial response is normal, the urinary osmolality should be 800–1400 mOsm/kg after dehydration, and a urine osmolality greater than 750 mOsm/kg effectively rules out diabetes insipidus. However, the urine osmolality should always be related to the plasma osmolality, since, if the latter is below 285–290 mOsm/kg, there is an inadequate stimulus to vasopressin release. Urine osmolality below 300 mOsm/kg that rises to above 750 mOsm/kg following vasopressin indicates cranial diabetes insipidus, whereas an absent response suggests nephrogenic diabetes insipidus. Patients whose plasma osmolality starts below 275 mOsm/kg may have psychogenic polydipsia, and it is important to ensure that such patients are adequately dehydrated before vasopressin is given; vasopressin administration to a patient whose plasma osmolality is subnormal is dangerous, and may cause fits. In difficult cases where the diagnosis remains unclear, hypertonic saline infusion followed by direct measurement of plasma vasopressin is possible in some centres. Such studies will also demonstrate the *sensitivity* of the osmolar-stimulated vasopressin system, its *threshold,* and the *thirst* threshold.

Treatment of Diabetes Insipidus

It is possible with currently available drugs to reduce the 24 h urine volume to below 2 litres and to render most patients with central diabetes insipidus virtually symptom free. This can be achieved in nearly every patient by replacing the hormone deficiency with vasopressin or one of its analogues, although, in cases with mild diabetes insipidus, control may be achieved through the use of non-hormonal agents such as chlorpropamide. Such drugs can either potentiate the action of otherwise inadequate quantities of endogenous vasopressin, e.g. chlorpropamide, or stimulate release of the hormone from the neurohypophysis, e.g. carbamazepine. Thiazides directly impair renal excretion and may be useful alternatives to vasopressin substitution therapy, but are generally reserved for patients with nephrogenic diabetes insipidus. Control of symptoms may be achieved with non-hormonal agents used singly or in combination. If control with such agents is unsuccessful, or if there is concern, for example, over the hypoglycaemic effects of chlorpropamide, then hormone replacement therapy should be used instead.

A major problem with the use of native vasopressin for treatment is its rapid inactivation, with a half-life in plasma of around 8 min. Until recently, intramuscular injections of pitressin tannate were used in the treatment of diabetes insipidus. The material was prepared from bovine pituitaries and the preparation had a longer antidiuresis than the native hormone, but the repeated injections were troublesome. A preparation of synthetic lysine vasopressin was then made available; this was administered as a nasal spray as the hormone is easily absorbed through the nasal mucosa; however, it frequently caused hypersensitivity reactions.

Many hundreds of analogues of neurohypophysial hormones have been synthesised, and recently a number of analogues have been produced of possible clinical value. These include preparations with reduced susceptibility to enzymic degradation and prolonged activity, with relatively selective pressor or antidiuretic effects. The antidiuretic action of vasopressin may be prolonged by removal of the N-terminal group and D-arginine substitiution at position 8. This also leads to a marked reduction in pressor activity, the resulting analogue, desamino-8-D arginine vasopressin (desmopressin, DDAVP) having selective antidiuretic activity. The antidiuretic action is also sufficiently prolonged that the hormone need only be administrered intranasally once or twice a day, and the doses used are well below the threshold for the pressor response or stimulation of vascular smooth muscle.

DDAVP has revolutionised the treatment of diabetes insipidus, although the intranasal insufflation technique may be difficult to learn. A measured amount of DDAVP (preferably via an insulin syringe) is inserted into a plastic cannula, and the liquid is blown into the anterior nares briskly while the patient sniffs. A metered-dose nasal spray is equally effective, but has not as yet been marketed. Most patients with complete cranial diabetes insipidus require 5–10 μg (5–10 μl) once or twice daily; if twice daily therapy is given, intermittent exclusion of a dose will allow for a diuresis of any possible water overload. It is important that the patient realises this, as the physiological excretion of excess fluid may be wrongly ascribed to poor control of the diabetes insipidus and the dose of DDAVP increased. Most recently, it has been realised that DDAVP is absorbed orally, although doses of the order of 100 μg 8-hourly may be required. However, this may obviously be of use in certain patients, especially children. A parenteral form is also available: 1 μg intramuscularly is approximately equivalent to 10 μg intranasally.

Other Uses for Vasopressin Analogues

Since it was first made available for treatment of diabetes insipidus it has been found that DDAVP can be used in the treatment of a variety of non-endocrine conditions. It has been used successfully in Von Willebrand's disease and moderately severe haemophilia A. In 1903 it was observed that the clotting time was accelerated in dogs following administration of adrenaline, and it was subsequently found that the vasoactive agents adrenaline and vasopressin could produce such an effect by elevating factor VIII activity. DDAVP has also been found to possess fibrinolytic activity, causing an increase in plasminogen activity and as well as in all components of the factor VIII system. It probably acts through release of a second messenger system, which in turn causes the release of factor VIII from its vessel-wall endothelial storage sites. Another potential use of DDAVP is in sickle-cell anaemia, a disease in which erythrostasis occurs. The red cells sickle owing to the formation of tactoids, or crystal-like fibres, from the polymerisation of deoxyhaemoglobin molecules. The tendency of the cells containing sickle haemoglobin to assume the sickle shape depends primarily on the concentration of intracellular deoxyhaemoglobin S. Since the red cells behave as osmometers, it follows that sickling may be decreased in a hypotonic solution. Although oral and intravenous hydration are used in the treatment of a sickle-cell crisis, it is difficult to produce a controlled state of hyponatraemia. This is now possible if the patient takes DDAVP and 3500–4000 ml water daily.

Another vasopressin analogue used clinically is triglycyl-lycine-vasopressin, a long-acting analogue with enhanced vascular activity. This analogue potentially may be used in the prevention of haemorrhage, e.g. from bleeding oesophageal varices or post-partum haemorrhage. The splanchnic area is particularly sensitive to the action of vasopressin, so infusions of vasopressin have been used in the reduction of bleeding from the gastro-intestinal tract. The hormone has been infused either intravenously or intra-arterially via the mesenteric arteries. Antagonists of vasopressin may prove to be of use in the treatment of SIADH, although full-scale clinical trials have not as yet been published.

As already indicated, analogues of vasopressin, including DDAVP, have been said to decrease memory disturbance in patients with Korsakoff's syndrome, and it has been suggested that central vasopressinergic pathways are involved in information processing. However, the effects are slight, and it has been suggested on the basis of animal studies that the changes produced are secondary to non-specific arousal.

Further Reading

Baylis, P.H. (1983) 'Posterior Pituitary Function in Health and Disease', *Clinics in Endocrinology and Metabolism, 12,* 747-70

Forsling, M.L. (1983) *Antidiuretic Hormone, Vol. 5*, Eden Press, Montreal

Forsling, M.L. (1985) 'Regulation of Oxytocin Secretion', in G. Ganten and D.P. Pfaff (eds), *Current Topics in Neuroendocrinology, Vol. 6, Neurobiology of Oxytocin,* Springer, Berlin

Manning, M., Grzonka, Z. and Sawyer, W.H. (1981) 'Synthesis of Posterior Pituitary Hormones and Hormone Analogues', in C. Beardwell and G.L. Robertson (eds), *Clinical Endocrinology, 1: The Pituitary,* pp. 265-96, Butterworths, London

Robinson, A.G. (1984) 'The Contribution of Measured Secretion of Neurophysin to our Understanding of Neurohypophysial Functions, in S. Reichlin (ed.) *The Neurohypophysis: Physiological and Clinical Aspects,* pp. 65-93, Plenum, New York

Zerbe. R., Stropes, L. and Robertson, G. (1980) 'Vasopressin Function in the Syndrome of Inappropriate Antidiuresis', *Annual Review of Medicine, 31,* 315-28

13 PITUITARY TUMOURS

Large pituitary tumours are uncommon tumours of the central nervous system and constitute approximately 10 per cent of all such tumours. The discovery of prolactin as a hormone distinct from growth hormone in 1970–71 led to the realisation that many chromophobe adenomas of the pituitary were actually prolactin-secreting tumours. This has had important clinical and therapeutic consequences, as will become clear. However, the measurement of serum prolactin has also led to the discovery of an increasing number of patients with small pituitary tumours — microadenomas — which cause hyperprolactinaemia but are unassociated with the effects of large space-occupying lesions (such as field defects, severe headache, hypopituitarism) which have been classically associated with lesions of the pituitary. Such microadenomas have become a common clinical problem quite distinct from the large tumours, and need to be discussed separately.

Pituitary Microadenomas

Natural History

Various histological studies have suggested that a large minority of the normal population have pituitary microadenomas. Such studies suffer from a number of defects, including poor definition of 'normality' and an absence of detailed endocrine data, but do suggest that pituitary microadenomas are a frequent autopsy finding. In one of the most comprehensive studies, 22 per cent of an unselected autopsy population were found to have such microadenomas, of which half the tumours were found to be positively immunostaining for prolactin. There is evidence that secretion of prolactin from tumours increases the delivery of hypothalamic dopamine into the portal vessels, suppressing the normal lactotroph population; thus a tumour will need to have a prolactin secretion rate greater than that of the normal pituitary before hyperprolactinaemia is produced. Nevertheless, it is likely that hyperprolactinaemia secondary to a prolactin-secreting microadenoma — a small prolactinoma — is a common clinical problem. In spite of the equal sex incidence at autopsy, patients presenting with symptoms secondary to small prolactinomas are usually female. As previously noted (see Chapter 7) such patients may present with oligomenorrhoea, amenorrhoea, regular cycles with a defective luteal phase, galactorrhoea, or symptoms of oestrogen deficiency, particularly superficial dyspareunia. This latter symptom is a frequent concomitant of hyperprolactinaemia, but may only be established on active enquiry by the clinician. Many such patients never come to medical attention as the symptoms may not be sufficiently severe to cause the patient any distress. In other cases, the oral contraceptive pill will produce regular withdrawal bleeds and suppress galactorrhoea and thus mask the symptoms of hyperprolactinaemia. Only a small proportion of patients with 'post-pill amenorrhoea' actually have hyperprolactinaemia, and there is currently no evidence that the use of the oral contraceptive has increased the evidence of small prolactinomas. It seems likely that patients with such tumours were diagnosed as having hypothalamic amenorrhoea or unexplained infertility before the introduction of the prolactin assay.

Radiologically, the pituitary fossa of patients with small prolactinomas may be completely normal, but small 'blisters' on its margin or sloping of the fossa floor (best seen on anteroposterior views) may be indicative of a tumour. However, analysis of a large series of plain skull radiographs in patients with small tumours did not show any precise correspondence between the presence and site of a tumour and a fossa abnormality, so that slight abnormalities would be interpreted with care. Conventional CT scanning is equally profitless, as these tumours rarely have suprasellar extensions. Nevertheless, the newer fourth and fifth generation CT scans with programs for sagittal and coronal reconstructions frequently demonstrate small intrasellar lesions only a few millimetres in diameter in patients with small prolactinomas. These are usually hypodense, but may be of varied consistency. Isodense lesions may sometimes be apparent, as the normal pituitary is pushed upwards causing a rather swollen pituitary to bulge upwards and distort the diaphragma sellae into forming a convex upper border. Although it has been claimed that all such tumours are visualised by means of the new CT scanners, it should be noted that many 'normal' subjects also have abnormal pituitary scans. It is possible that such subjects are harbouring clinically-inapparent microadenomas, but there is also a case to be made that so many so-called microadenomas are functionless cysts. Only a large-scale correlative study comparing endocrine data with surgical findings will ultimately settle this uncertainty.

Many tests have been devised to distinguish the small prolactinoma from so-called 'functional hyperprolactinaemia', which is envisaged as a functional derangement in the control of prolactin secretion. In normal subjects serum prolactin rises after the administration of TRH, or the dopamine antagonists metoclopramide or domperidone; serum prolactin falls after nomifensine, an antidepressant which blocks dopamine uptake in the hypothalamus and thus increases its availability to the portal vessels. Patients with small prolactinomas have blunted prolactin responses to TRH, metoclopramide and domperidone, and show little fall in prolactin after nomifensine. Patients with functional hyperprolactinaemia are said to respond more like normal subjects. However, there are many false positives and false negatives associated with the use of every test so far devised, and responsiveness generally correlates inversely with the serum prolactin in patients with histological evidence of tumours as well as those with 'functional hyperprolactinaemia'. Most authorities consider that the great majority of patients with hyperprolactinaemia have small prolactinomas so that the serum prolactin may merely be measured on several occasions in the absence of any dynamic function tests. The only method of settling this controversy is to correlate normal and abnormal dynamic function tests with surgical outcome, as was discussed in relation to CT scanning. However, surgeons are understandably reluctant to operate on patients in whom the standard tests are said not to indicate the presence of tumours.

Apart from hyperprolactinaemia, endocrine function in patients with small prolactinomas is generally normal. The high serum prolactin decreases the release of LHRH from the hypothalamus, resulting in inhibition of pituitary gonadotrophin release. Basal levels of gonadotrophins are generally normal, but in about one-third of patients the gonadotrophin response to LHRH is exaggerated. This may reflect an increase in the readily releasable pool of LH and FSH consequent upon their diminished release. In a similar proportion of patients, the TSH response to TRH is also enhanced. The reason for this is uncertain, but may relate to the fact that hyperprolactinaemia increases the portal delivery of dopamine. A clearer demonstration of this phenomenon is revealed by the enhanced TSH response to dopamine antagonists in patients with hyperprolactinaemia. Although it has been suggested that this enhanced response is only seen in patients with prolactinomas, careful examination of the published data shows a correlation between this response and the serum prolactin in all patients with hyperprolactinaemia. As these tumours do not typically have suprasellar extensions, visual fields are usually normal. Diabetes insipidus is not a feature of pituitary microadenomas.

The aetiology of small prolactinomas remains unknown, with no evidence that the oral contraceptive is important in provenance. Lactotrophs are scattered throughout the normal pituitary but the tumours are preferentially located in the lateral wings of the gland. This has fuelled speculation that the tumour may start as a small clump of cells which is disconnected from the portal capillaries by a microvascular occlusion. Those cells near to the border of the gland may avoid infarction by developing a new vascular supply from capsular branches of the hypophysial arteries. As the peripheral vascular system has only low levels of circulating dopamine, this clump of cells may be stimulated to undergo hypertrophy, hyperplasia and possibly adenomatous transformation.

Treatment

There has probably been no area of greater controversy in modern neuroendocrinology than over the treatment of small prolactinomas. Part of the problem has been the paucity of information regarding the natural history of the condition, and therefore the uncertainty as to whether the outcome of a course of treatment is actually secondary to that treatment. Nevertheless, in the last few years, sufficient data has been amassed to enable reasonable guidelines for therapy to be suggested. There is little doubt that, untreated, most small prolactinomas do not significantly change in size or secretion rate. Such patients can be reassured that they are unlikely to develop large pituitary tumours, and treatment should be planned bearing this in mind. In a few patients serum prolactin falls with time, sometimes to within the normal range, although this is unusual. Equally, in the occasional case the small prolactinoma may continue to grow, with a rise in serum prolactin. It is therefore important that all patients, even if untreated, are reviewed at yearly or two-yearly intervals with a check skull radiology and serum prolactin assessment.

For the majority of patients, the probable treatment of choice is dopamine agonist therapy. Most experience has been gained with bromocriptine, but newer agents, such as pergolide or sustained-release bromocriptine, may allow the convenience of once-daily treatment. The dose is gradually built up, always being taken in the middle of food, until serum prolactin is normalised. This will lead to cessation of the galactorrhoea and a resumption of normal menses, irrespective of the length of the preceding amenorrhoea. Fertility should also rapidly return. In the case of patients presenting with amenorrhoea and infertility, it is reasonable practice to advise the couple to use mechanical contraception until the woman has had two or three regular menstrual cycles. In the absence of contraception, delay in menses for more than two or three days usually indicates conception, most conveniently confirmed by a sensitive serum hCG estimation. The bromocriptine can then be stopped, as there is no evidence in the human (unlike the rat) that prolactin is involved in the maintenance of the corpus luteum. Extensive world-wide experience has so far suggested that conceptions achieved by means of bromocriptine have no higher incidences of multiple births or congenital malformations than occur in the normal population. However, it is sensible to stop bromocriptine at the earliest opportunity.

An initial fear was that pregnancies in patients with small prolactinomas would induce tumour enlargement, causing headache and field defects, secondary to oestrogen stimulation of the adenoma. Fortunately, this seems rarely to occur (probably in less than 1 per cent of cases), although some physicians would advise regular monitoring of the visual fields during pregnancy. Post-partum there is anecdotal evidence that breast-feeding is associated with a relatively high incidence of breast abscess formation and some women are reluctant to breast-feed. If the woman does decide to breast-feed, it is reasonable to monitor her carefully for signs of breast engorgement in the early stages.

Most data suggest that when bromocriptine is stopped, the serum prolactin returns to its pretreatment level. This implies that therapy, when required, may need to be continued for many years. For patients to whom this is unacceptable, or who are resistant to (or intolerant of) dopamine agonist therapy, an alternative mode of treatment is trans-sphenoidal microadenomectomy. This technique, originally developed by Harvey Cushing but considerably popularised by Jules Hardy, who introduced the operative microscope and preoperative screening, allows for selective removal of the microadenoma. The usual approaches are either transnasal or peroral, and in experienced hands the total operation time can be less than one hour. Some surgeons operate transethmoidally, but this leaves a scar alongside the bridge of the nose and is less cosmetically acceptable. Experience from several centres suggests that the *best* results represent an 85–90 per cent immediate cure rate, with normalisation of serum prolactin and retention of residual pituitary function. Transient diabetes insipidus may occur, but other hormone deficiencies are rare, as are the perioperative complications of CSF rhinorrhoea or meningitis. This approach to the treatment of small prolactinomas has been particularly espoused in North America, where the introduction of bromocriptine was delayed for many years by the FDA. Unfortunately, the cure rate falls off noticeably as the serum prolactin rises, especially above the 4000 mU/litre. Furthermore, the very good results are only obtained by surgeons with extensive training and special expertise in such surgery.

Most troublesome is the question of recurrence. One series suggests that up to 50 per cent of small prolactinomas treated surgically may recur at 5 years. Although this is not universally agreed, there is as yet little published information on the long-term results of surgery. Whether or not the return of hyperprolactinaemia truly indicates tumour recurrence may be considered academic, as the patient will still require treatment, but there is evidence that prolactin dynamics are rarely normalised even with a normal serum prolactin postoperatively. Perhaps the most reasonable approach to the treatment of small prolactinomas, based on current evidence, is to use dopamine agonist therapy in the first instance. More than 90 per cent of patients will respond with a normalisation of serum prolactin with minimal side-effects. Patients intolerant of one dopamine agonist may respond better to a different drug, but true resistance to bromocriptine (which may need to be given in a dose of up to 60 mg/day) usually generalises to other drugs. Patients who are resistant to or intolerant of dopamine agonists should be offered the possibility of trans-sphenoidal surgery, preferably in a major centre. Reluctance to be on long-term medication is another possible indication for surgery, although patients have been on bromocriptine for up to 15 years with no evidence of long-term side-effects.

Finally, should hyperprolactinaemia always be treated? There is accumulating evidence that the oestrogen deficiency secondary to hyperprolactinaemia may actually cause osteoporosis, and even in the short term, normalisation of serum prolactin may produce an improvement in libido, sexual enjoyment and dyspareunia. However, the truly asymptomatic patient with a normal plasma oestradiol may simply be observed, especially if menstruating, albeit intermittently.

Oestrogen-containing oral contraceptives should never be given to the untreated patient with a prolactinoma, as this may induce tumour growth and expansion. In a small series of patients, one study suggested that such oral contraceptives could be used in patients whose prolactin had been normalised by means of bromocriptine. However, close supervision is required.

Microadenomas secreting ACTH or GH will be dealt with later in this chapter.

Pituitary Macroadenomas

Macroadenomas are pituitary tumours greater than 1 cm in diameter. They may be associated with local pressure effects, including expansion of the pituitary fossa causing headache, and upward extension to compress the visual pathways, and cause field defects, lateral extension into the cavernous sinuses or beyond (giving rise to facial pain, abnormalities in eye movement, or temporal lobe dysfunction), or inferior extension and herniation through the sphenoid sinus into the back of the nose. Although such tumours are only extremely rarely truly malignant, metastasising to other parts of the central nervous system and beyond, local invasion is not uncommon. The tumours do not have true capsules, but may compress the surrounding tissue into a dense band as a 'pseudocapsule'. Hormonal

178 *Pituitary Tumours*

effects may occur, either as a result of direct tumour secretion or secondary to tumour disruption of the normal pituitary and its connections with the hypothalamus (Figure 13.1).

Figure 13.1: Scheme for Classification of Pituitary Tumours

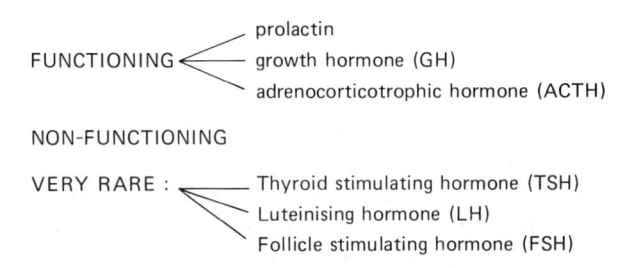

```
                        prolactin
         FUNCTIONING    growth hormone (GH)
                        adrenocorticotrophic hormone (ACTH)

         NON-FUNCTIONING

         VERY RARE :    Thyroid stimulating hormone (TSH)
                        Luteinising hormone (LH)
                        Follicle stimulating hormone (FSH)
```

Prolactinomas

Although 60–70 per cent of pituitary tumours may be associated with hyperprolactinaemia, only about 40 per cent are true prolactinomas, i.e pituitary tumours immunostaining for prolactin and assumed to be actively secretory. Such tumours are usually chromophobe adenomas, but may occasionally be eosinophilic (Figure 13.2). Electron microscopy reveals the presence of prolactin secretory granules, although individual cells are usually sparsely granulated. Women may present with symptoms and signs of hyperprolactinaemia, as with small prolactinomas, but may in addition have evidence of local pressure effects or hypopituitarism. Men with hyperprolactinaemia are much more likely to have a large prolactinoma and may present with erectile failure secondary to hyperprolactinaemia; however, they are more likely to seek medical attention because of field defects or other local effects. In children, GH deficiency will lead to a failure of growth, and in young people of either sex, hyperprolactinaemia may produce delayed or arrested puberty.

Serum prolactin is usually above 2500mU/ml in these patients, but may be two to three orders of magnitude higher. There is a rough correlation between the size of the tumour and the level of serum prolactin, such that large tumours associated with a serum prolactin below 2500 mU/litre are unlikely to be prolactinomas. Tumour expansion initially leads to growth hormone deficiency, but in adults this can only be detected by an inadequate growth-hormone response to a stimulation test, usually the insulin tolerance test (ITT). Loss of the gonadotrophins then occurs, followed finally by loss of ACTH reserve and the development of secondary hypothyroidism. Diabetes insipidus is rare, and if detected suggests the presence of a primary hypothalamic tumour such as a craniopharyngioma or a germinoma. Plain skull radiology will generally show a large ballooned fossa, but the full extent of the tumour is best outlined by high-resolution CT scanning. Pituitary fossa tomography is rarely required nowadays, and pneumencephalography or metrizamide/iopadol cisternography is reserved for difficult

Figure 13.2: Light Microscopy of a Prolactinoma (A) before, and (B) after, Immunostaining for Prolactin Using the Immunoperoxidase Technique. (Courtesy of Professor I. Doniach.)

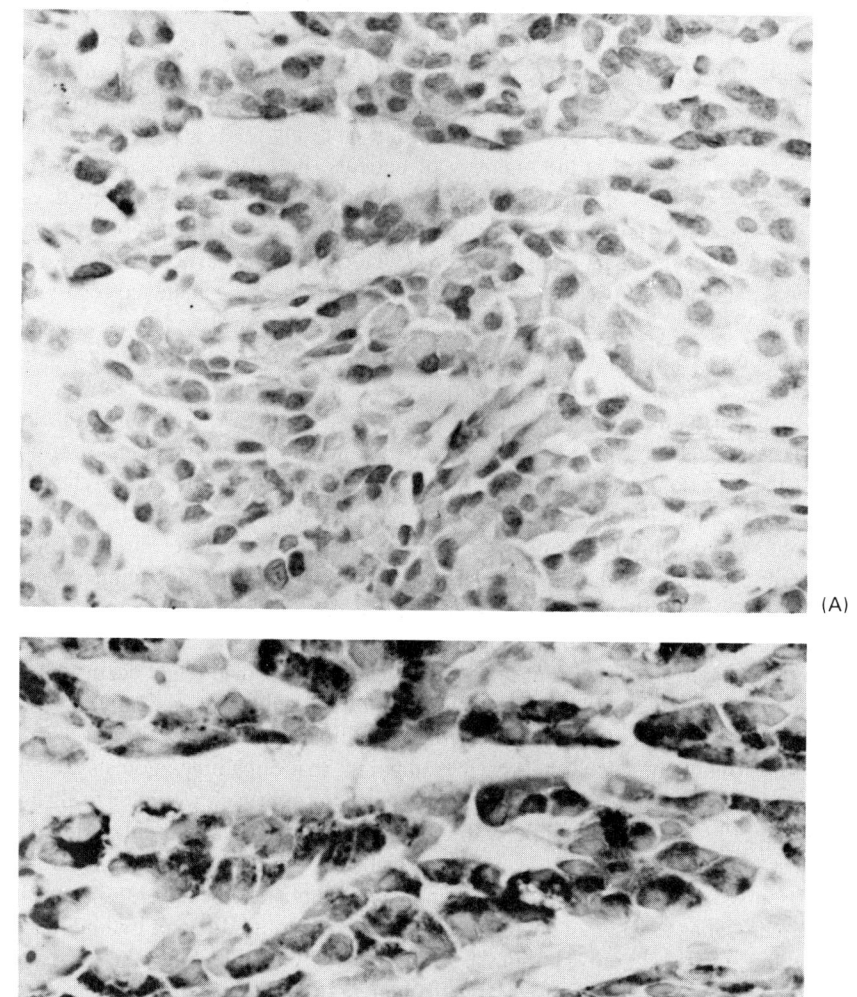

(A)

(B)

cases, such as differentiation of an empty fossa (*vide infra*) from a cystic tumour. Angiography is usually only necessary to exclude a carotid aneurysm, or to establish the anatomy before transcranial surgery. Field defects are highly variable: bitemporal hemianopia is classical but not typical, and may only be recorded by testing in very dim lighting. Quadrantic field defects in the lower temporal fields usually indicate a compressive lesion from above, i.e. a hypothalamic tumour.

Dopamine agonist therapy of such tumours not only leads to a normalisation of the serum prolactin in the majority of patients, but also produces shrinkage of at least 80 per cent of tumours. Field defects improve, often within a few days, and residual endocrine function may also improve. An injectable depot formulation of bromocriptine, has recently been developed, and is particularly useful in such patients, as it allows blood levels of bromocriptine to be achieved relatively easily and rapidly. Detailed histological studies have demonstrated a considerable diminution in cell size in prolactinomas so treated, with loss of cytoplasm and a decrease in granular endoplasmic reticulum. Initially, secretory granules increase in density as exocytosis diminishes, but eventually a decrease in prolactin synthesis, as well as release, produces a decrease in secretory granules and possibly a loss in prolactin immunostaining. Prolactin cell number does not seem to change, although recently reports of cell necrosis and fibrosis have appeared. On long-term treatment, tumour shrinkage and prolactin eventually level out, although cases of 'escape' from therapy have been reported. Cessation of dopamine agonist treatment is usually associated with a gradual rise in serum prolactin and re-expansion of the tumour, so bromocriptine is best considered as tumorstatic rather than tumorcidal. In some instances, symptomatic re-expanison may occur within a few days, whereas in other patients the tumour may only very gradually regrow. The reasons for these differences are unclear, but may relate to the preceding length of treatment. Nevertheless, it is apparent that dopamine agonists cannot be considered to represent definitive treatment. One approach would be to shrink the tumour as much as possible with dopamine agonists, and thereafter attempt trans-sphenoidal removal. This is usually feasible so long as the tumour has shrunk sufficiently so as to leave no more than a small suprasellar extension. There is disagreement as to whether such surgery is rendered more difficult by long-term dopamine agonist therapy, but in the short term there is little doubt that tumours previously only amenable to a transfrontal craniotomy can now be tackled transsphenoidally. Postoperative radiotherapy can then be used to prevent tumour recurrence. It should be noted that tumour shrinkage may be asymmetric, and this, together with the increased fibrosis that may occur (rendering operative removal difficult), suggests that the radiotherapy field should encompass the size of the *original* tumour.

An alternative approach is to use external beam radiotherapy alone as tumorcidal therapy for prolactinomas that have been shrunk away from the optic chiasma by dopamine agonist therapy. This treatment produces a gradual fall in serum prolactin over several years and may allow for the eventual discontinuation of dopamine agonists (Figure 13.3). Hypopituitarism does not seem to be a problem in the medium term (4–5 years), and replacement therapy is rarely required at follow-up times ranging up to 10–12 years. Macroprolactinomas are liable to swell during pregnancy and although the risk may not be as high as the previously reported 25 per cent, it is still sufficient of a problem to determine treatment policy. External beam radiotherapy allows pregnancy safely to be undertaken without risk of tumour expanison and in the knowledge that the requirement for long-term bromocriptine use will diminish and eventually disappear. Using 4500 cGy as a total dosage, delivered by three fields at a daily dose of less than 200 cGy, visual pathway damage, radionecrosis or radiation-induced tumour are extremely uncommon. However, the long-term incidence of hypopituitarism remains unknown, and the patient should be followed up for life.

Figure 13.3: The Effect of External Radiotherapy on Serum Prolactin in Patients with Prolactinomas. Reproduced from Grossman et al. (1984),'The Treatment of Prolactinomas with Megavoltage Radiotherapy', *British Medical Journal, 288,* 1105-9 by permission of the authors and the Editor of the *British Medical Journal*

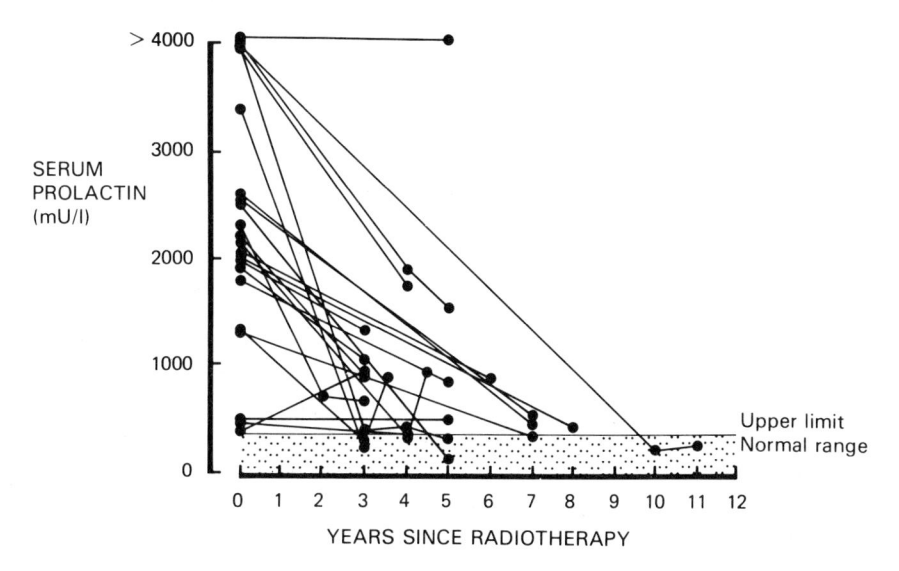

Large prolactinomas without significant suprasellar extensions may be treated by the same means, although some authorities consider that dopamine agonists alone are an effective definitive treatment. Any evidence of tumour expansion during pregnancy can then be treated by reinstituting bromocriptine or a related drug, a procedure which has so far been shown to be safe and effective. There is certainly evidence that such tumours may occasionally greatly improve post-partum, with a lowering or normalisation of serum prolactin. Measurement of serum prolactin during pregnancy is not particularly helpful, although a value in excess of 10 000 mU/litre should alert the clinician to the possibility of an expanding lesion.

Internal radiotherapy with yttrium implant appears to prevent pregnancy-induced tumour expansion and may lead to long-term tumour regression. However, the technique is available at few centres and rarely normalises serum prolactin.

Patients presenting with hyperprolactinaemia and an enlarged pituitary fossa may have the 'empty fossa syndrome' with CSF herniating into the fossa and leaving the normal pituitary as a thin rim around the fossa floor. Some of these cases may represent tumour infarcts, and patients may sometimes give a history of severe headaches and neck stiffness that spontaneously resolve. In other cases, particularly where the rest of the pituitary is functioning normally, a congenital defect in the diaghragma allows CSF gradually to fill the fossa and compress the normal pituitary. In neither case does treatment extend beyond normalisation of the serum prolactin, where this is thought to be clinically appropriate. A frequent problem is the asymptomatic patient who has plain skull radiology following minor trauma and is then found to have a ballooned pituitary fossa. History and examination are usually normal, as is endocrine testing including serum prolactin measurements. If a high-resolution scan reveals an empty fossa, no action is required other than reassurance. Follow-up at prolonged intervals may be advisable, although there is little evidence that such lesions progress to endocrine deficiency.

Functionless Tumours

Approximately 30 per cent of pituitary tumours are functionless in that they are not thought to secrete any of the known hormones. The presence of secretory granules in the cells of such tumours is of unknown significance. Although serum prolactin may be normal, not uncommonly it may be raised due to tumour disruption of the hypophyseal portal system. The hyperprolactinaemia due to these 'pseudoprolactinomas' is usually slight (less than 1500 mU/litre), but levels up to 6000–8000 mU/litre have occasionally been reported. Patients with such tumours usually present with field defects, headache, or symptomatic hypopituitarism — particularly changes in menstrual pattern in women or poor libido and erectile failure in men. These tumours do not significantly shrink with dopamine agonist therapy, and surgery followed by prophylactic radiotherapy is necessary. In the patient presenting with a large pituitary tumour and a serum prolactin between 1500 and 8000 mU/litre, a trial of dopamine agonist therapy to shrink a presumptive prolactinoma may be instituted. Frequent assessment of visual fields and acuities is mandatory. A field deficit persisting after a short course of such treatment with no significant tumour shrinkage demonstrable radiologically indicates the need for early surgery.

Occasionally patients with 'functionless tumours' are found not to have adenomas, but rather functionless cysts such as an epidermoid cyst or Rathke's pouch cyst. Intrasellar craniopharyngiomas are also seen, and may or may not be associated with diabetes insipidus or intrasellar calcification. Pituitary calcification may also indicate a 'pituitary stone', presumably an infarcted pituitary tumour or the rare 'idiopathic pituitary fibrosis' (a variant of the midline fibrosing syndrome).

Cushing's Disease

In most patients with pituitary-dependent Cushing's syndrome there is a basophil adenoma of the pituitary. However, the tumour is usually small, and in 90 per cent of patients plain skull radiology shows either a normal fossa or minimal asymmetry. As the microadenoma may be isodense and difficult to distinguish from normal tissue, CT scanning is not always helpful. Local pressure effects or hypopituitarism are rare, other than the hormonal effects due to the high circulating level of cortisol (see Chapter 11). Where the clinical and biochemical evidence is clearly in favour of pituitary-dependent Cushing's syndrome, especially when confirmed by a venous catheter with petrosal sinus sampling for ACTH, transsphenoidal surgery is both diagnostic and therapeutic. The tumours usually lie medially or posteromedially, often clearly apposed to the posterior pituitary. Successful microadenomectomy is followed by acute cortisol deficiency, as the normal corticotrophs have been suppressed by the elevated circulating corticosteroids. It is reasonable to treat the patient with metyrapone for several weeks prior to surgery to reduce perioperative complications such as wound infections. Diabetes insipidus may occur, but it is usually transient; other evidence of hypopituitarism is variable unless the surgeon has attempted a total fossa clearance for a larger, more aggressive tumour. If there is no evidence of ACTH deficiency immediately post-operatively, many authorities would probably advise prophylactic radiotherapy to avoid the development of Nelson's syndrome. Steroid replacement therapy may be necessary for periods ranging from a few months to several years after surgery. Histologically, most tumours are basophil or chromophobe adenomas immunostaining for ACTH; sometimes normal corticotrophs are also removed and these may show the typical Crooke's change (hyaline cells due to filamentous deposition in the cytoplasm) characteristic of corticosteroid excess. Although some centres have reported a subset of tumours showing multifocal sites of 'pars intermedia' cells, it is uncertain how common such tumours really are. However, it is undoubtedly true that not infrequently no adenoma can be found, with histology suggestive of corticotroph hyperplasia. It has been suggested that this is secondary to excess CRF secretion. Hypothalamic gangliocytomas may also secrete CRF and cause pituitary-dependent Cushing's syndrome.

Possibly 90 per cent of patients with Cushing's disease are cured by transsphenoidal microadenomectomy, and this remains the treatment of choice. External beam or yttrium radiotherapy are second-line treatments and may take some years to control the disease. They are useful in the therapy of recurrent or incompletely removed tumours; metyrapone can be used for interim control of cortisol levels.

There are few indications nowadays for bilateral adrenalectomy. Such patients require life-long corticosteroid replacement therapy and the tumour remains *in situ*. There is thus the high risk of Nelson's syndrome arising (approximately 20–30 per cent of patients) unless radiotherapy to the tumour is also given. Occasionally, it is difficult to remove the right adrenal from the inferior vena cava, and following ACTH stimulation the adrenal remnant regrows to produce a true recurrence of Cushing's syndrome. However, study of such adrenalectomised patients has been extremely useful in understanding the cause of pituitary-dependent Cushing's syndrome: the most carefully conducted studies suggest that all of the endocrine associations of this syndrome (attenuated TSH responses to TRH and growth-hormone responses to hypoglycaemia, etc.) are a consequence purely of the steroid excess. They provide little evidence in favour of a primary hypothalamic derangement.

An expanding pituitary tumour secreting ACTH may arise *ab initio* or may be stimulated following bilateral adrenalectomy for Cushing's disease (Nelson's syndrome). Radiotherapy to the pituitary should certainly be used if bilateral adrenalectomy is the primary mode of therapy, but it is uncertain whether it can prevent all cases of Nelson's. The combination of surgery and radiotherapy may not be effective for some of the more particularly aggressive ACTH-secreting tumours. Occasional tumours respond to dopamine agonists such as bromocriptine with a fall in ACTH levels, but in our experience these are rare. Cyproheptadine, an antiserotoninergic drug, has been reported to normalise ACTH levels in up to a third of patients with pituitary-dependent Cushing's syndrome, but the effect is unreliable and the drug is sedative and causes a considerable increase in appetite. *In vitro* data suggest that it may directly interfere with the tumour cells' secretory machinery, rather than interacting with serotonin receptors. Sodium valproate increases GABA levels and may control secretion of ACTH; both it and cyproheptadine are probably best reserved for patients with Nelson's syndrome, as these tumours may offer a considerable therapeutic problem.

Some 'functionless' tumours may immunostain for ACTH, probably representing a corticotroph tumour of limited secretory capacity. There is at least one recorded case of such a tumour presenting as a functionless tumour and recurring to cause the full clinical syndrome of Cushing's disease.

Acromegaly

By contrast to Cushing's disease, the majority of tumours associated with excess growth hormone secretion are macroadenomas and are usually apparent with plain skull radiology. Suprasellar, lateral or sphenoidal extensions are not uncommon. Although some of the smaller tumours can be successfully removed transsphenoidally, larger tumours will require radiotherapy to sterilise the residual tumour. An alternative approach is to assess the bromocriptine sensitivity of serum growth hormone levels, and where bromocriptine leads to normalisation or near normalisation of serum growth hormone, external radiotherapy can be given as definitive treatment. Periodic withdrawal of bromocriptine (or its equivalent) will allow for assessment of residual tumour secretion. Hypopituitarism is more common following radiotherapy to these tumours as opposed to prolactinomas, but in about 70 per cent the mean serum growth hormone is below 10 mU/litre at ten years (Figure 13.4). Radiotherapy is more often effective when serum GH levels are only moderately elevated. The advent of somatostatin therapy may increase the response of such tumours to medical treatment and therefore increase the use of radiotherapy (Figure 13.5). It should also be noted that bromocriptine itself may lead to tumour shrinkage, even in the absence of hyperprolactinaemia (*vide infra*). However, primary treatment for bromocriptine-unresponsive tumours remains trans-sphenoidal surgery, followed, when appropriate, by radiotherapy.

Figure 13.4: Serum Growth Hormone in Patients with Acromegaly Treated by External Radiotherapy. (Courtesy of Dr J.A.H. Wass.)

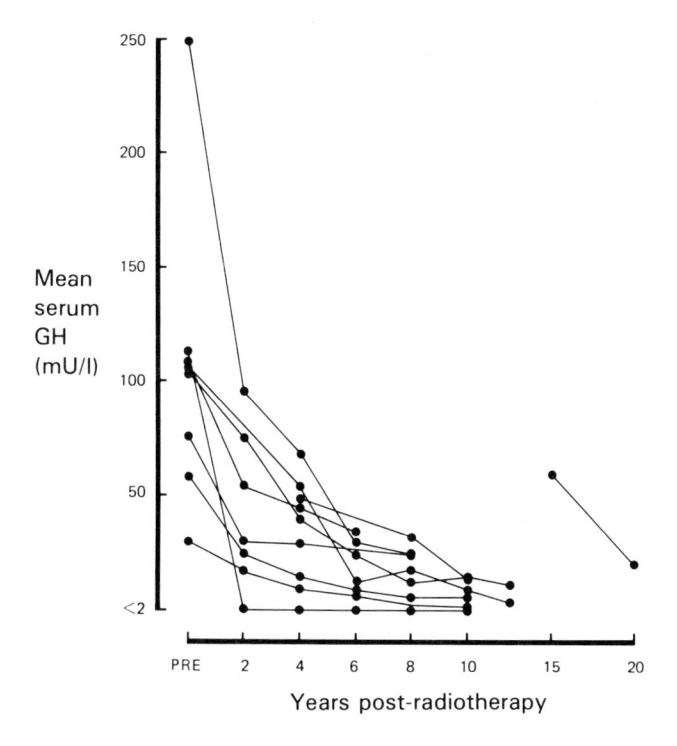

Hyperprolactinaemia occurs in one-third of patients with acromegaly. This may be due to interference with the hypophyseal-portal vasculature, but true tumour secretion is also seen. Separate cells may secrete prolactin and growth hormone, or the same cell (the somatomammotroph) may secrete both. The so-called 'stem cell' tumour is characterised by hyperprolactinaemia, low but non-suppressible levels of growth hormone, and a rather aggressive growth pattern.

In the instance of patients with acromegaly, it has been suggested that many do not require treatment except on cosmetic grounds. However, it has now been decisively demonstrated that acromegaly decreases life expectancy, even if the local pressure effects of the tumour are excluded. Even small tumours can have a high secretory capacity and be associated with hypertension, diabetes mellitus and a cardiomyopathy. Nevertheless the tumour may also be slow-growing, with photographic evidence over many decades of growth-hormone hypersecretion.

Figure 13.5: Plasma Growth Hormone in Eight Patients with Acromegaly Infused with Somatostatin (GH-RIH, 500 µg). Longer-acting analogues are currently under trial. (Courtesy of Dr J.A.H. Wass.)

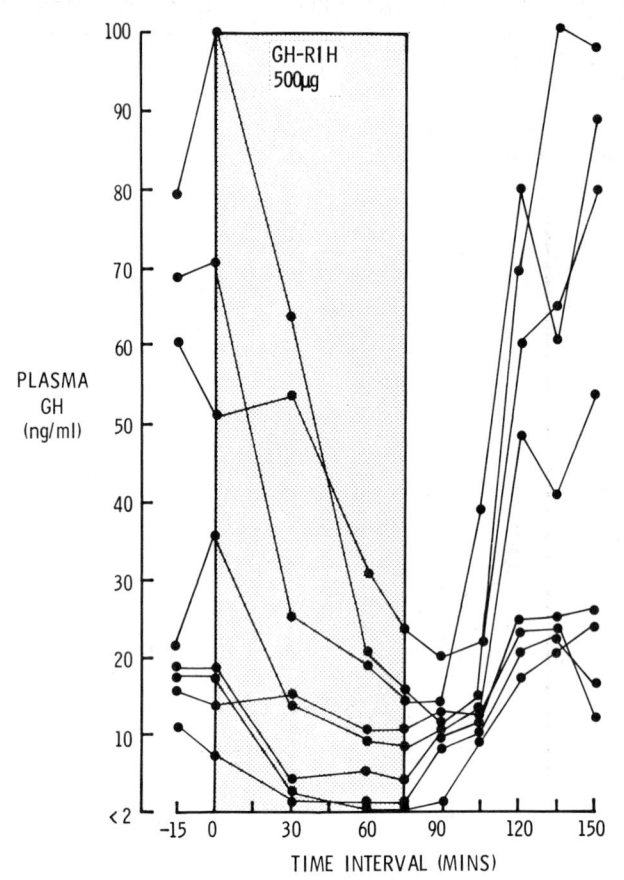

Under these circumstances, it is evident that an immediate and complete normalisation of growth-hormone levels may not be essential. Indeed, there is considerable argument as to what constitutes a cure in acromegaly. Some authorities consider that patients with mean serum GH levels of less than 5, 10 or even 20 mU/litre are 'cured', whereas others may require an absent GH response to TRH in addition. Some even requre that serum GH become undetectable during a standard glucose tolerance test in a 'cured' patient. It is clear that taking the most strict criteria, few patients are ever completely cured.

In the young patient with a microadenoma, trans-sphenoidal surgery is probably the treatment of choice. Although many such patients are left with low levels of serum growth hormone (10 mU/litre), abnormal responses to TRH frequently remain. The decision as to whether to employ postoperative radiotherapy will depend on the surgical ease of removal and the postoperative mean level of serum growth hormone, but should probably be the exception rather than the rule. In older patients, especially where the tumour is large with a significant extrasellar extension, bromocriptine may be used as a trial to assess the response of the tumour, both in terms of size and secretion, to dopamine agonist therapy. An improvement in symptoms and a marked fall in serum growth hormone may allow radiotherapy to be given safely with interim dopamine agonist therapy. It should be emphasised that in acromegaly bromocriptine needs to be given four times daily, so that newer, long-acting preparations such as pergolide (allowing adminstration two to three times a day) are preferable. Massive tumours may be shrunk away from the optic chiasma by dopamine agonist therapy followed by external radiotherapy. When shrinkage does not occur — a rather more common finding than with prolactinomas — trans-sphenoidal or occasionally transfrontal surgery followed by radiotherapy is necessary. Radical removal in this instance is not curative and is more likely to cause serious neurological damage. As mentioned above, improvements in medical therapy are likely to improve the ability to control growth-hormone hypersecretion and thus avoid surgery. However, definitive treatment is still necessary in all but the very frail patients or the mildest cases.

Acromegaly and Carcinoids

As described in Chapter 8, there are patients with pancreatic or bronchial carcinoids secreting GHRH who present with acromegaly. Such patients cannot be diagnosed as having ectopic GHRH secretion from the clinical or endocrine features of the acromegaly. Serum growth hormone responses to glucose, insulin, TRH or exogenous GHRH are unhelpful. Measurement of circulating GHRH is most useful as the levels in such patients are many orders of magnitude higher than in normal subjects (in such normal subjects the low level of circulating GHRH probably derives from the gut or pancreas). However, studies of circulating GHRH in several hundred patients with acromegaly have demonstrated ectopic GHRH secretion causing acromegaly to be a very rare syndrome.

The Clinical Approach to the Patient with a Pituitary Tumour

In approaching the patient with a possible pituitary tumour, as in all clinical medicine, the history and examination are vital. In children, evidence of a failure to thrive or to grow are paramount, but will not be evident in adults. A detailed sexual history is particularly important, as early symptoms of changes in libido in men and women, erectile failure in men, or irregular menses in women are significant early findings. Symptoms due to changes in the pituitary, thyroid and pituitary-adrenal axes are relatively subtle, and may merely present as general fatigue, weakness, or a slowing up. Diabetes insipidus is initially most evident to the patient as nocturia, but the polydipsia that goes with polyuria may most concern the patient. Field defects may be present for a surprisingly long time without obvious symptoms, but eventually patients will notice their tendency to bump into things. A complete bitemporal hemianopia will cause the interesting

Figure 13.6: Suggested Scheme for Pituitary Hormone Replacement Therapy. Oral DDAVP may soon be clinically available

ANTERIOR PITUITARY

Thyroxine	0.2 mg daily (check T_3)
Hydrocortisone	20 mg mane, 10 mg at 18.00 (check cortisol day curve)
Sustanon or Primoteston	500 – 750 mg i.m. 2 – 6 weekly
OR	
Ethinyl oestradiol + Medroxyprogesterone acetate	30 µg daily 5mg daily 1st 7 days of each month

POSTERIOR PITUITARY

DDAVP	10 – 20 µg intranasally at night (check plasma and urine osmolality)

phenomenon of postfixation blindness: if a patient with such a defect is asked to focus on a given object, for example a pencil, he will suddenly find he is unable to see any object behind that pencil. The headache associated with pituitary tumours has no special characteristic feature, but in the absence of hydrocephalus it is rarely associated with papilloedema or vomiting. A careful drug history is essential, as many tranquillising drugs as well as antiemetics may cause hyperprolactinaemia.

The examination should particularly be orientated towards the sexual anatomy, and evidence of hypogonadism must be sought. A change in body hair, diminution in size or consistency of the testes, or a soft feminisation of the skin are sometimes seen in male patients. In the female, evidence of change in breast size should be sought, and particularly galactorrhoea. Although it has been claimed that only one-third of women with hyperprolactinaemia do have galactorrhoea, this percentage considerably increases if it is carefully looked for. Testing for field defects with an 8 mm red pin is specially recommended, as subtle defects are occasionally only manifest by a change in the intensity of the red colour of the pin. In some cases an early field defect is only manifest originally as temporal desaturation to red, i.e. the red pin looks brighter in the nasal as compared to the temporal visual field. In addition, testing in dim lighting will sometimes bring out a mild defect.

Baseline endocrine tests should always be carried out before more dynamic testing. These should include basal serum thyroxine, a plasma cortisol between 08.00 and 09.00, a basal plasma testosterone level in men and oestradiol in women, and circulating gonadotrophins and prolactin in both sexes. A paired early-morning plasma and urine osmolality should also exclude patients with gross diabetes insipidus. Dynamic endocrine screening can then be considered as appropriate (see Chapter 14). In patients with suspected Cushing's syndrome, an overnight dexamethoasone suppression test will produce few false negatives and may be used as a screening test. In cases of suspected acromegaly, an out-patient glucose tolerance test with measurement of blood glucose and growth hormone may be all that is required.

Radiological assessment of patients with pituitary tumours has changed considerably in recent years. A good-quality plain lateral and postero-anterior skull radiograph is still useful, but fossa tomography and pneumo-encephalography are now seldom required. Access to a high-resolution CT scan is almost mandatory for the proper care of all such patients. In terms of treatment, replacement therapy for each axis of the pituitary must be considered. A suggested schema for a typical patient with panhypopituitarism is given in Figure 13.6. However, it should be noted that replacement must be tailored to each individual's requirements on the basis of clinical and biochemical responses. In childhood, GH therapy must also be considered.

Further Reading

Belchetz, P.E. (1984) *Management of Pituitary Tumours,* Chapman & Hall, London
Black, P.M., Zervas, N.T., Ridgway, E.C. and Martin, J.B. (1984) *Secretory Tumors of the Pituitary Gland,* Raven Press, New York
Givens, J.R. (1982) *Hormone-secreting Tumours,* Year Book Medical Publishers, Chicago
Beardwell, C. and Robertson, G.L. (1981) *The Pituitary,* Butterworths, London
Camanni, F. and Muller, E.E. (1984) *Pituitary Hyperfunction,* Serono Symposium 10, Raven Press, New York
Faglia, G. Giovanelli, M.A. and Macleod, R.M. (1980) *Pituitary Microadenomas,* Proceedings of Serono Symposium 29, Academic Press, London

14 NEUROENDOCRINE TEST PROCEDURES

As indicated in the earlier chapters, an underlying endocrine disease may not be immediately apparent and, indeed, ideally should be detected before the clinical features of that disease have become advanced. The symptoms result from excess secretion or underactivity, which may be established by hormone estimations. Since basal secretion of pituitary hormones is pulsatile, estimation of plasma hormone levels is not necessarily discriminatory and suppression and stimulation tests may have to be performed. Such tests may also indicate the site of a particular lesion, be it in the hypothalamus, pituitary or target organ. Tests of hypothalamic function are listed in Table 14.1 and are described in detail in this chapter.

Table 14.1: Dynamic Tests of Hypothalamo — Pituitary Function

Disorder	Test
Growth hormone deficiency	Insulin tolerance (ITT); glucagon; standardised exercise; GHRH;
Acromegaly	Glucose tolerance test
Hypothalamic-pituitary-adrenocortical axis	
Hypofunction (Addison's disease)	Short adrenal stimulation test
Pituitary insufficiency	Insulin tolerance; CRF
ACTH oversecretion	Metyrapone; dexamethasone; CRF; Insulin tolerance
Hypothalamo-pituitary-gonadal axis	
Hypothalamic reserve	Clomiphene stimulation test
Pituitary reserve	LHRH stimulation test
Gonadal (testicular) failure	hCG
Hypothalamo-pituitary-thyroid axis	
Pituitary function	TRH test
Posterior pituitary function	
Pituitary vasopressin	Water deprivation test; hypertonic saline infusion

The Insulin Tolerance Test

The insulin tolerance test (ITT) has been the mainstay of neuroendocrine testing for the past 15 years, and looks likely to remain so. Its principal use lies in testing the dynamic reserve of the pituitary-adrenal and growth-hormone axes, but it is also useful in the diagnosis of Cushing's syndrome. The essence of the test is the induction of neuroglycopenia as a 'stress' which activates hypothalamic neurones to stimulate (ultimately) the release of ACTH and GH.

In terms of the pituitary-adrenal axis, hypoglycaemia is thought to release CRF, which in turn stimulates the release of plasma ACTH and hence cortisol. For most purposes, only circulating cortisol is usually measured. It has been shown that if circulating cortisol rises above a peak level of 550 nmol/litre, then no corticosteroid cover is necessary for any major stress, including surgery. It is possible that peak cortisol levels around 600 nmol/litre may still be associated with a partial deficiency of CRF or ACTH, but this is not clinically significant. A subnormal cortisol response to hypoglycaemia suggests a deficiency in either CRF or ACTH production or release — a CRF test can then be used to locate precisely the biochemical level of the lesion (see below). For marginally subnormal responses, e.g. a peak cortisol in the range 400–550 nmol/litre, the patient may only need corticosteroid treatment during acute illness or operation; lower levels require that the patient be given hydrocortisone replacement therapy. In the diagnosis of Cushing's syndrome, a normal circulating cortisol that fails to rise with hypoglycaemia is highly suggestive of the diagnosis; a normal cortisol response is seen in the pseudo-Cushingoid syndrome of depressive illness.

Hypoglycaemia also stimulates GH release, almost certainly via an increase in GHRH. Peak GH levels above 20 mU/litre generally exclude any major abnormality, although ususally much greater responses are seen. Borderline responses are occasionally seen in the peripubertal period, and may be normalised by 'priming' with gonadal steroids. The ITT is a more sensitive test than exercise testing, and is generally in greater use than stimulation with amino acids such as arginine or ornithine. Some authorities consider that clonidine, and adrenoceptor α-agonist, is a safer and equally reliable stimulus to GHRH release, but this test is of very little use in the post-childhood age group. However, it is possible that the ITT and clonidine tests do not assess exactly similar parameters, as the results are not always concordant. Recent studies suggest that there is a close concordance between the GH response to an ITT and the nocturnal peak of GH.

Procedure

An intravenous cannula is inserted into the forearm of the supine patient between 07.30 and 09.00, the patient having fasted from midnight. Insulin 0.15 U/kg is administered as an acute bolus 30 mins later, and blood is taken basally and at 30-minute intervals (plus 45 minutes) for 2 h for cortisol, GH, and blood sugar. Hypoglycaemia occurs at 20–30 min and peak GH and cortisol levels at 45–120 min. The patient should be closely monitored throughout, and symptoms of neuroglycopenia (palpitations, perspiration) recorded. If uncertain as to whether hypoglycaemia is present, rapid glucose recording of a venous sample with a digital-read-out glucose meter may be helpful. The patient may be drowsy, but should not be allowed to sleep. Fifty millilitres of 50 per cent dextrose should be kept drawn up and within reach and administered immediately should the patient become unrousable, start twitching, or have an epileptic fit. If this proves necessary, blood sampling should still be continued (if possible) to the end of the test. Intravenous hydrocortisone should also be available. At the termination of the test, a glucose drink such as 'Lucozade' should be given, followed by a substantial meal. The patient should not be discharged home until he or she feels completely well and until at least 2 h have elapsed since the completion of the test. The patient should be on bed-rest throughout, and should not be allowed to sleep at any time during the test or for 2 h thereafter.

Precautions

No patient with a history of epilepsy, ischaemic cardiac test, or cardiac dysrhythmia should have an ITT. All patients should have a basal 09.00 cortisol, serum thyroxine, and ECG some time before the test, and the ITT must be cancelled if any of these is abnormal. A basal cortisol at 09.00 of less than 180 nmol/litre usually indicates a deficiency in the pituitary-adrenal axis, necessitating steroid replacement therapy. If it is still considered necessary to carry out an ITT on such a patient, corticosteroids should be given for some time prior to the test to increase hepatic glycogen stores. (Glucagon and, to a lesser extent, catecholamine mobilisation of glycogen stores are the principal counter-regulatory responses to hypoglycaemia. A failure to appreciate this fact led to early fears regarding the safety of the ITT, which are now known to be groundless if proper precautions are taken.) In children, 0.10 U/kg of insulin is usually sufficient to induce hypoglycaemia. In patients with suspected glucose intolerance (e.g. acromegaly, Cushing's syndrome), an initial dose of insulin 0.3 U/kg may be used. If symptoms of neuroglycopenia are absent, and blood monitoring does not confirm hypoglycaemia, a further dose of 0.15 U/kg may be given and sampling recommended as before.

Criteria for Normality

If the minimum blood glucose is less than 2.2 nmol/litre, and symptoms of neuroglycopenia are present, then circulating cortisol and GH increase to > 550 nmol/litre and > 20 mU/litre, respectively in normal subjects.

The Glucagon Test

In older patients, or the very young (< 5 years of age), or in those with pre-existing cardiac or cerebral dysrhythmias, a glucagon test may replace the ITT. The procedure is as above, except that glucagon is given rather than insulin (1 mg *subcutaneously*, or 1.5 mg subcutaneously in patients weighing more than 90 kg); samples are taken at 0 and 90 mins, and then every 30 mins for 2½ h. and sampling is continued for 4 h. The test is less sensitive and specific than the ITT, and its mechanism of action is unknown. It was originally thought that glucagon increased blood glucose, and that the eventual decline in blood glucose to basal levels was responsible for the stimulation of cortisol and GH release. However, the test is subjectively unpleasant and often induces nausea and vomiting, such that it may function as a non-specific stressor. The same careful observation is required as for the ITT. Although a normal response to glucagon is helpful, a poor or absent response may not necessarily be pathological. Some authorities consider that in childhood a glucagon dose of 0.1 mg/kg, given intramuscularly rather than subcutaneously, increases the sensitivity and usefulness of the test without increasing side-effects.

Metyrapone has also been used as an alternative test of cortisol reserve. However, as cortisol feeds back at both hypothalamic and pituitary levels, a rise in cortisol in response to metyrapone does not guarantee a normal hypothalamo-pituitary-adrenal axis.

The TRH Test

TRH stimulates the readily releasable pool of pituitary TSH, and can be used as a test of pituitary TSH reserve or as an indirect test of peripheral thyroid hormone effects.

Procedure

An intravenous forearm cannula is inserted into the patient in the morning, and a bolus of TRH 200 µg is administered. Blood is taken for serum TSH, at 0, 20 and 60 min. The test is best performed in the morning, as there is a circadian rhythm in TSH secretion, but fasting is unnecessary. Bed rest is advisable but not essential.

Side-effects

Most patients experience a transient feeling of perineal tightening or an urge to micturate, and they should be warned about this. Occasional nausea or facial flushing may also be noted, but are rarely severe. Very rarely, TRH administration is associated with severe headache, and there are also case reports of pituitary infarction following TRH. It is possible that these are idiosyncratic hypertensive crises induced by TRH, which should never be given to such patients on a second occasion.

Interpretation

In normal subjects with normal circulating T_4 and T_3 levels, TRH causes a transient rise in TSH at 20 min, with a partial fall to baseline at 60 min. An absent TSH response to TRH is seen in thyrotoxicosis, but can also be present in patients with multinodular goitres. Patients with primary hypothyroidism usually have elevated basal levels of serum TSH, with exaggerated responses to TRH; in borderline primary hypothyroidism, a normal serum TSH may also respond excessively to TRH. In the presence of a frankly subnormal serum T_4, a serum TSH that is not elevated suggests that the cause of the hypothyroidism lies in the pituitary or hypothalamus. In such instances, a delayed response to TRH, with the 60-min TSH greater than the 20-min sample, suggests hypothalamic disease; an absent TSH response to TRH in such patients indicates pituitary failure, while an apparently 'normal' response is unhelpful.

Attenuated TSH responses to TRH may be seen in patients on corticosteroids, and in those with depressive illness, renal failure, or Parkinson's disease. Enhanced responses may be seen in hypoadrenal patients. Patients with thyrotoxicosis, in association with high circulating levels of TSH that do not respond to TRH, may have TSH-secreting pituitary adenomas.

TRH also induces a rise in serum prolactin in normal subjects. Blunted or attenuated responses are seen in hyperprolactinaemic patients, especially if this is secondary to a prolactinoma. However, absent prolactin responses to TRH may also occasionally be seen in normal subjects.

A 'paradoxical' GH response to TRH may be seen in acromegaly, chronic renal failure, hepatic failure, and anorexia nervosa.

The LHRH Test

LHRH stimulates the readily-releasable pool of LH and, to a lesser extent, FSH. However, there are a number of circulating substances that feed back at the pituitary level, including testosterone and inhibin in males, and oestrogens, progesterone and inhibin in females. Thus the gonadotrophin response to GnRH may be highly variable, even in the same woman at different times of the menstrual cycle.

Procedure

An intravenous forearm cannula is inserted into the patient: the time of day is not critical, and fasting is unnecessary. However, the day of the menstrual cycle should be noted in menstruating women, and comparisons should always be made within the same phase, e.g. early or midfollicular. A bolus of 100 μg LHRH is given, and blood is sampled at 0, 20 and 60 min.

Side-effects

The test is safe and without side-effects; bed-rest is not required.

Interpretation

In men, a low basal testosterone in association with elevated gonadotrophins which respond excessively to LHRH is indicative of primary hypogonadism. A subnormal testosterone level in association with a normal serum LH is indicative of hypothalamo-pituitary disease; the gonadotrophin response to LHRH does not allow the level of the abnormality to be localised. Similarly, normal gonadotrophin levels in women with subnormal plasma oestradiol levels, or in women obviously post-menopausal, is pathological, but LHRH testing does not usually add further information. In patients with prolactinomas, there may be normal, subnormal or even enhanced gonadotrophin responses to LHRH. The presence of normal or enhanced LH and FSH responses to LHRH in amenorrhoeic patients with hyperprolactinaemia usually suggests that such patients will menstruate once their hyperprolactinaemia is treated.

Poor or absent gonadotrophin responses to LHRH are seen in prepubertal children, or in patients with anorexia nervosa. Normal responses to LHRH, often with a relatively enhanced FSH response, precede the outward manifestations of pubertal onset. LHRH may induce an increase in serum prolactin during the luteal phase in normal women, and very occasional patients with acromegaly may respond to LHRH with a rise in serum GH.

The CRF Test

CRF-41 is available as a synthetic peptide from several sources, although the purity of preparations may differ. At the time of writing it is only available for clinical research and in a few centres, but may become more widely available in the future. Both human (hCRF) and ovine (oCRF) CRF-41 are available. Although most experience has been obtained with oCRF-41, recent studies have suggested that the actions of hCRF-41 are similar to those of oCRF-41, albeit slightly shorter in duration.

Procedure

Following overnight fast, the patient has an intravenous cannula inserted for blood sampling and drug administration. CRF-41 is usually dissolved in acid saline to minimise adsorption to syringe, tubing, etc., and is given as an intravenous bolus at a dose of either 1 μg/kg, or a standard dose of 100 μg. Blood is sampled for cortisol, and ACTH and related peptides if desired, for 2 to 3 hours.

Side-effects

Flushing occurs in about 20–30 per cent of patients, but is usually transient. Severe hypotension and arrhythmias have been reported, but are extremely uncommon at the doses given. Nevertheless, monitoring of blood pressure and pulse would be wise, and availability of resuscitation equipment is mandatory.

Interpretation

Every laboratory needs to establish its own normal range for cortisol responses to CRF-41. Published studies suggest that responses are independent of age and sex. Generally speaking, in a patient with little or no cortisol response to an ITT, a normal response to CRF-41 suggests a defect in the production or release of endogenous CRF, or in its access to the pituitary via the portal vasculature. In patients with suspected Cushing's syndrome, a greatly enhanced cortisol response outside of the normal range strongly suggests pituitary-dependent Cushing's syndrome. An absent response to CRF-41 suggests an ectopic rather than a pituitary source of ACTH in documented Cushing's syndrome. Normal patients with high basal levels of cortisol respond poorly to CRF-41. Patients with depressive illness and dexamethasone-resistant cortisol levels respond to CRF-41 like normal subjects.

The GHRH Test

Similar considerations apply to GHRH as for CRF-41. Synthetic GHRH (1–44) NH_2, GHRH (1–40) and GHRH (1–29) NH_2 are available for clinical research only at present, but will almost certainly become more widely available in the near future. The three peptides are approximately equipotent. Normal ranges need to be defined independently for each unit or hospital, and are age-dependent. The most important use of the GHRH test is in defining the site of the lesion in adult patients with subnormal GH responses to ITT, or in children with subnormal responses to an ITT or clonidine test (Figure 14.1). The procedure and dosage are identical to that for CRF-41. Mild flushing may occur, but more serious side-effects have not been reported. Attenuated GH responses to GHRH may also be seen in non-fasted patients, obese patients, the elderly, and in adults with long-standing GHRH deficiency.

Figure 14.1: Levels at which the Insulin Tolerance Test (ITT) and Growth Hormone Releasing Factor (GRF) Stimulate Growth Hormone Release

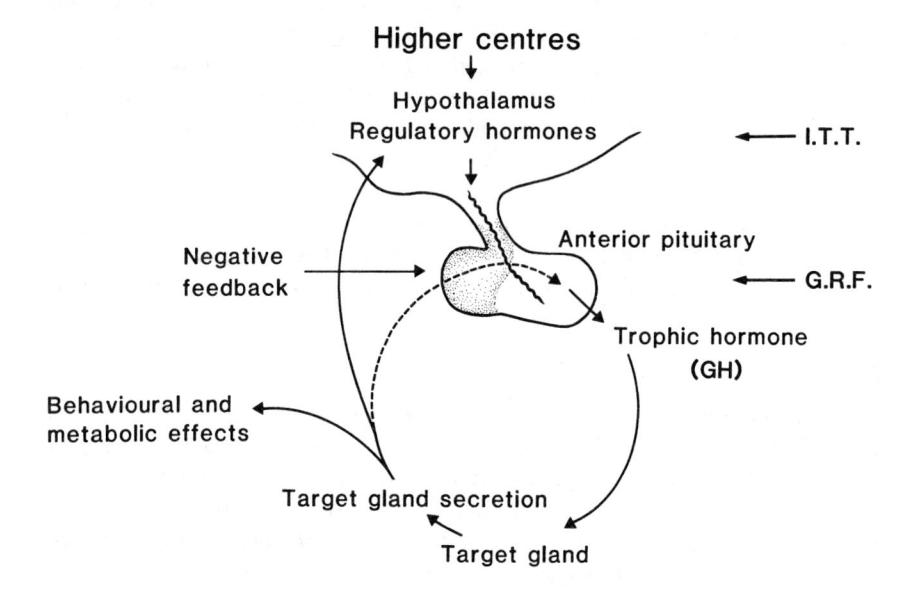

Combination Tests

TRH, LHRH and the ITT may be administered concurrently, which is of considerable advantage in the investigation of the patient with hypopituitarism. However, both hypoglycaemia and TRH stimulate prolactin release, such that measurement of serum prolactin in the combined test is rarely helpful. TRH and LHRH may also be combined with CRF-41 and GHRH; in this instance there is evidence that GHRH may enhance the TSH response to TRH, but the effect is slight and may not be clinically significant. It should be noted that CRF-41 and GHRH cannot replace the ITT, as the former tests the readily releasable pituitary reserve whereas the ITT assesses the hypothalamo-pituitary axis. The former should therefore be considered as complementary test procedures.

The Clomiphene Test

Clomiphene is an oestrogen with mixed agonist-antagonist properties, which is principally used as an oestrogen antagonist to stimulate the release of hypothalamic LHRH. In normal subjects, a ten-day course of clomiphene (50 mg tds; if weight < 50 kg, 50 mg bd) will double serum LH and FSH levels, or produce a rise to outside the normal range. Although there has been recent evidence that clomiphene may act, at least in part, at the level of the pituitary, an absent response to clomiphene in conjunction with a normal response to LHRH generally suggests a hypothalamic defect. Such responses are particularly seen in Kallman's syndrome, weight-loss-related menstrual problems, and anorexia nervosa. In severe cases of LHRH deficiency, clomiphene may actually act as an oestrogen agonist and suppress gonadotrophin levels. Poor responses to both clomiphene and LHRH do not help in localising gonadotrophic defects. Patients should be warned that clomiphene may cause side-effects such as flushing, depression, or visual anomalies such as flashing lights. These may be briefly disturbing but are rarely severe.

Prolactin Stimulation Tests

As discussed in Chapter 7, tests relying on the stimulation of prolactin by pharmacological agents to discriminate prolactinomas from functional hyperprolactinaemia are rarely of much clinical use. Where there is suspected prolactin deficiency, e.g. in a patient with Sheehan's syndrome, serum prolactin may be measured during a standard TRH test.

The Dexamethasone Suppression Test

In normal subjects, dexamethasone 0.5 mg 6-hourly for 48 h leads to a suppression of urinary 11-hydroxycorticosteroids. The dexamethasone should be given at exact time intervals, i.e. at 09.00, 15.00, 21.00 and 03.00, and the patient should be warned that the drug may cause insomnia. Although originally defined in terms of urinary corticosteroids, recent data suggest that a serum RIA cortisol below 180 nmol at 48 h also indicates normality. Failure of suppression is seen classically in Cushing's syndrome, but may also occur in depressive illness and in alcoholic pseudo-Cushing's. The test may also be used to investigate the adrenal dependence of androgen secretion: in women with the polycystic ovary syndrome, elevated serum testosterone, androstenedione and the dehydroepiandrosterone sulphate usually fall to within the normal range with dexamethasone.

High-dose dexamethasone (2 mg 6-hourly for 48 h) will cause a 50 per cent or greater fall in urinary corticosteroids in patients with pituitary-dependent Cushing's syndrome, but not in patients with Cushing's syndrome due to other causes. However, in this instance its principal use is in differentiating ectopic from pituitary causes of excess ACTH secretion, although the differentiation is not absolute.

The overnight dexamethasone test is of low accuracy. However, if only a relatively low dose of dexamethasone is used, it can be used to *exclude* the great majority of patients with suspected Cushing's syndrome. One milligram is given at midnight, and serum cortisol is measured between 08.00 and 09.00. A level below 180 nmol/litre is seen in normals; a level above this requires that the patient be subjected to the full 48-h low-dose dexamethasone supression test.

The Metyrapone Test

In the metyrapone test, metyrapone 750 mg is given 4-hourly for six doses starting at 09.00. The tablets are always given in the middle of food, the minimum being a sandwich and a glass of milk. The patient should be advised to lie flat for the first 4 h, and mobilised gently at the end of 24 h. Serum cortisol falls acutely, causing an increase in ACTH release and hence in cortisol precursor metabolites in normal subjects and in patients with pituitary-dependent Cushing's syndrome. In other cases of Cushing's syndrome, urinary 17-ketogenic steroids rise to values less than twice the basal levels on the day of, or the day after, metyrapone administration. The patient needs to be on bed-rest for 24 h, and urinary collections must be exact. In this form, the test is of very poor discriminatory value. There is some evidence that a single 24-h measurement of serum 11-deoxycortisol is more useful in differentiating Cushing's disease (values > 1000 nmol/litre) from other causes of Cushing's syndrome.

Water Deprivation Test

The water deprivation test for neurohypophysial function is based on the premise that in normal subjects the maximum obtainable urine concentration is limited by the renal concentrating ability rather than on vasopressin release, which is the case in patients with diabetes insipidus. In normal subjects, dehydration produces a greater rise in urine osmolality than administration of DDAVP. Thus if, after dehydration, vasopressin administration induces a further increase in urine osmolality, vasopressin deficiency should be suspected. Under most circumstances careful measurements of the osmotic pressure of the plasma and urine provide an excellent way of diagnosing diabetes insipidus, and the renal response will adequately differentiate pituitary from nephrogenic diabetes insipidus.

Procedure

The water deprivation test must be carried out with careful supervision. Patients with pronounced vasopressin deficiency may become severely dehydrated, and compulsive water drinkers may attempt to drink during the test. Vasopressin release is influenced by a number of drugs including hypnotics, ethanol and nicotine, so that, if possible, drugs should be stopped (except steroid replacment therapy) and patients should not be allowed to smoke during the test. It is most convenient to start the test at 08.00 following a light breakfast without tea or coffee. Water only should be drunk before the test. Plasma and urine samples are collected for the determination of osmolality before the fast and at hourly intervals for 8 h. During this time the patient should have nothing to eat or drink. The fast should be terminated earlier if the patient's weight falls by 5 per cent or more. When either 8 h have elapsed or the plateau of urine concentration is reached (no change in successive urine samples greater than 30 mOsm/kg), DDAVP may be given in a dose of 2 μg or 20 μg intranasally, and further urine samples should be collected for 12 h. After the administration of DDAVP, the patient may have a light meal, but drink no more than twice the volume of urine passed during the fluid restriction.

Interpretation

Under normal conditions, urine osmolality should reach 600 mOsm/kg or more, with the plasma osmolality not rising above 300 mOsm/kg. In diabetes insipidus, plasma osmolality exceeds 300 mOsm/kg, with the urine osmolality remaining at less than 300 mOsm/kg. Pituitary diabetes insipidus may be confirmed by correction of urinary concentration with DDAVP. Unfortunately, patients may have intermediate responses, so the differential diagnosis between diabetes and overdrinking becomes difficult.

Hypertonic Saline Infusion

A more consistent means of achieving osmotic stimulation of vasopressin is probably by hypertonic saline infusion rather than fluid deprivation. However, direct measurement of plasma vasopressin is required as vasopressin secretion cannot be determined by following changes in urine osmolality and flow rate, because such changes are influenced by the natriuresis resulting from the sodium load.

Procedure

The patient is fasted overnight and only allowed to drink water before the start of the test. No smoking is allowed. The patient empties the bladder and is weighed. Two intravenous cannulae are inserted, one for sampling and the other for infusion, after which the patient rests supine for 30 min. Two basal blood samples for the estimation of plasma vasopressin and osmolality are taken with an interval of 10 min, and then 0.855 M NaCl (5 per cent saline) is infused at a rate of 0.06 ml/kg/min for 2 h. Blood pressure is recorded at 15-min intervals and

Figure 14.2: Vasopressin Response to Hypertonic Saline Infusion in Patients without Diabetes Insipidus (Panel A; A-D) and in Patients with Diabetes Insipidus (Panel B; E-J). Reproduced from Baylis, P.H. (1983), 'Posterior Pituitary Function in Health and Disease', in *Clinics in Endocrinology and Metabolism*, 12, pp. 747–70, with the permission of the author and the Editor of *Clinics in Endocrinology and Metabolism*

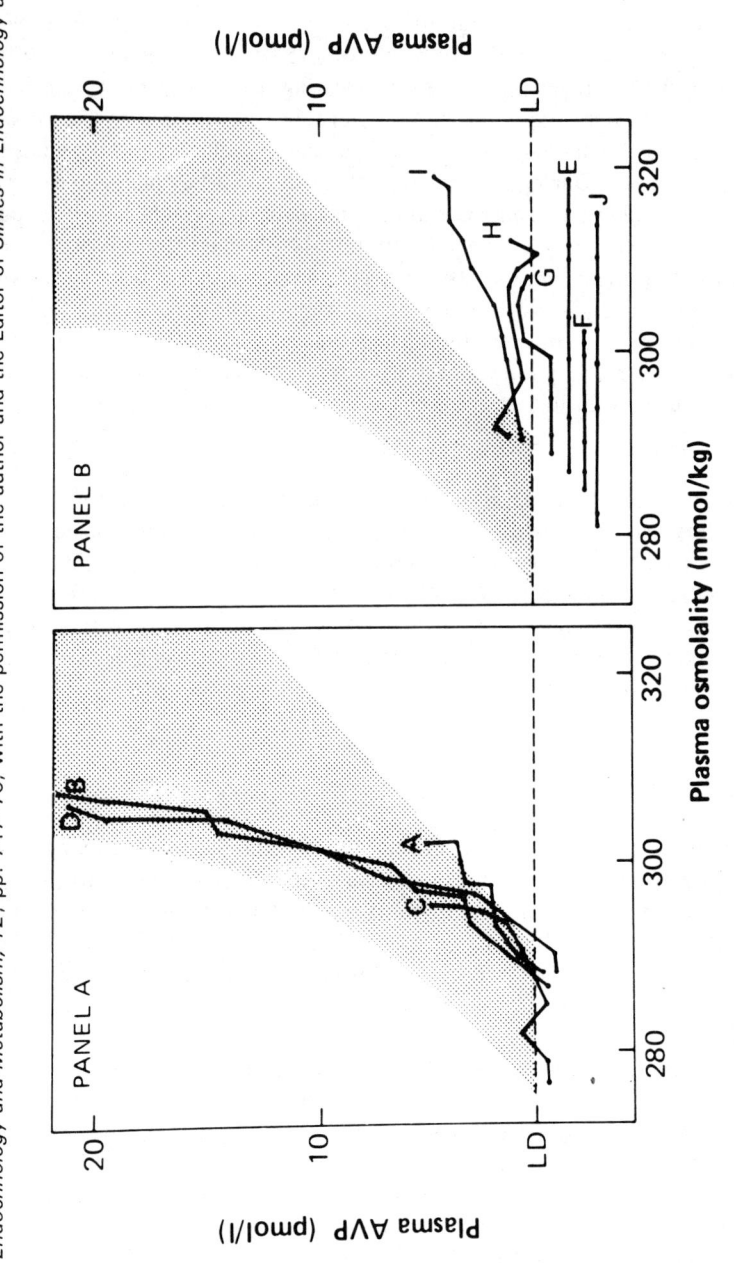

blood samples are taken at 30-min intervals, with a final sample 15 min after the end of the infusion. The time of onset of thirst is noted, and if the patient complains of severe thirst he or she may be given a few ice chips to suck. The patient may normally drink after the test, but should avoid rapid ingestion of large volumes of fluid.

Interpretation

With plasma osmolality in the normal range (275–290 mOsm/kg) there is considerable overlap of vasopressin concentrations in patients with cranial diabetes insipidus and others (see Figure 14.2). However, as plasma osmolality rises, separation becomes distinct, with little or no increase in plasma vasopressin being seen in patients with cranial diabetes insipidus. In patients with either primary polydipsia or nephrogenic diabetes insipidus, plasma vasopressin rises with osmolality. This test also allows for some evaluation of osmoreceptor function. Most patients report the marked sensation of thirst between 293 and 305 mOsm/kg, as do normal individuals. Infusion of hypertonic saline provides a method of distinguishing hypodipsic and adipsic patients, who often also have abnormalities in osmotic stimulation of vasopressin release.

Further Reading

Baylis, P.H. and Gill, G.V. (1984) 'The Investigation of Polyuria', *Clinics in Endocrinology and Metabolism, 13* 295–310

Crapo, L. (1979) 'Cushing's Syndrome; a Review of Diagnostic Tests', *Metabolism, 28,* 955–77

Hall, R., Anderson, J., Smart, G.A. and Besser, G.M. (1980) *Fundamentals of Clinical Endocrinology,* Pitman, London

Lamberton, R.P. and Jackson, I.M.D. (1983) 'Investigation of Hypothalamic-pituitary Disease', *Clinics in Endocrinology and Metabolism, 12,* 509–34

INDEX

Acetyl choline 56, 57
Acidophil 5, 6
Acromegaly 2, 28, 101, 184-7
Adenoma 73
Adenosine 3'5' monophosphate see cyclic AMP
Adenylate cyclase 63, 64, 67
Adrenal cortex 143-4
Adrenaline 63
Adrenergic neurones
   α-receptors 56, 57
   β-receptors 55, 57
Adrenocorticotrophin 5, 7, 12, 17, 28, 41, 47, 60, 135-45
Air encephalogram 180
Aldosterone 52
Amenorrhoea 119, 173
Ammonium sulphate 22
Amniotic fluid 12
Amygdala 38
Androgens 116-17, 188
Angiotensin II 31
Anorexia nervosa 118, 122, 194
Anterior commisure 4
Antibody 19-21, 65
Antidiuretic assay 16
Antidiuretic hormone see vasopressin
Appetite 32
Arachidonic acid 71
Arachnoid cyst 11
Arcuate nucleus 35
Arginine 42
Arginine vasopressin see vasopressin
Arginine vasotocin 11
Assay, bioassay 10-19, 76-7
   kits 29-30
   radioimmunoassay 20-30, 76-7
Autoimmune disorders 74
Axo-axonic interactions 1

Basophils 5
Behaviour 31
Bentonite 25
Beta endorphin 137-8
Binding reagent 21
Bioassay see assay
Biosynthesis 37, 38
Blood-brain barrier 54
Blood pressure 50
Brainstem 39

Bromocriptine 28, 83, 86-7, 103, 133, 151, 176

Calcium 53, 62, 64, 70-2, 131
Calmodulin 71
Carbamezepine 160, 168-9
Carrier-mediated transfer 73
Catalytic subunit (of protein kinase) 67
Cerebrospinal fluid 10, 44, 54
Charcoal 22
Childbirth 115, 165
Chlorpromazine 81
Chlorpropamide 168-9
Cholesterol 143
Cholinergic pathways 54, 140
Chordomas 44
Chromatography 28
Chromophils 5
Chromophobes 6
Circadian rhythms 31, 51, 92, 143
Clomiphene 41, 120, 196-7
Clonidine 59, 94, 105
Cold stress 56, 127, 130
Conception 114
Corpus luteum 114
Corticotrophin see adrenocorticotrophin
corticotrophin-like intermediate peptide (CLIP) 136
Corticotrophin releasing factor 3, 34, 41, 51, 57, 139-41, 194-5
Corticotrophs 6
Cortisol 52
Craniopharyngioma 10, 43
Cushing's disease 145-52, 183-4
   syndrome 28, 144-5
Cyclic AMP 53, 62-4, 67-72
   GMP 53, 70
Cyproterone acetate 123
Cytochemical assay 17-19, 138

DDAVP 170-1, 188
Dehydration 169
Delayed puberty 123
Dexamethasone 128, 142, 197-8
Diabetes insipidus 3, 32, 42, 43, 166
   mellitus 3, 145
Diaphragma sella 3
Diurnal rhythm see circadian rhythm
DNA (deoxyribose nucleic acid) 64
Dopamine 11, 34, 58, 59, 79-80, 83

203

Index

Dopaminergic pathways 54, 110, 128
Dose-response curve 19, 29
Down-regulation 66, 120
Drinking 31
Dura mater 3

Electron microscopy 6-7
Empty sella syndrome 11
Endorphin 137
Enzymes 62
Enzyme-immunoassay 20
Epidermoid cysts 10, 43
Exocytosis 33
Extraction (for assay) 25-6

Fatty acid 97
Feedback 1, 48-51, 58
Feeding 31
Fergusson's reflex 164
Fetus 5
Field defects 4, 187
Fluoro-immunoassay 20
Follicle stimulating hormone 5, 49, 108 *et seq.*
Fornix 38

GABA 60, 79, 140
Galactorrhoea 85
Gigantism 101
Glucagon 93, 192-3
Glycogen 63
Glycogenolysis 68-9
Glycoprotein hormones *see* LH, FSH, TSH
Gonadotrophin releasing hormone *see* LHRH
Gonads 12
Gonadotrophs 6
Grave's disease 74, 132, 193
Growth hormone 5, 8, 11, 15, 56, 90-7
Growth hormone release inhibiting hormone *see* somatostatin
Growth hormone releasing hormone 33, 56, 99-100, 187, 195-6
Guanyl diphosphate 68
Guanyl triphosphate 68

Habenular nucleus 38
Haemorrhage 159
Half-life 77
Hamartomas 45, 120
Hashimoto's thyroiditis 74
Herring Body 9
High performance liquid chromatography (HPLC) 29
Hippocampus 38
Histamine 60, 130, 140
Histiocytosis 43

Hodgkin's disease 84
Horse-radish peroxidase 6
Huntington's chorea 80
5-hydroxytryptamine 11, 39, 94, 130, 140, 156
Hyperphagia 42
Hyperprolactinaemia 40, 59, 82-8
Hypoglycaemia 60, 190-1
Hypogonadism 120-2
Hypopituitarism 178, 188
Hypothalamic hormones 33-4, 40, 46, 51, 53 *see also individual hormones*
Hypothalamic nuclei 37
Hypothalamus 31-46
Hypothyroidism 83, 132
Hypophysectomy 3, 176-7

Immunoabsorbant 23
Immunocytochemistry 6
Immunofluorescence 6
Immunoradioimmunoassay 23, 26-8
Infertility 82, 118, 120
Infundibulum 3, 5
Inhibin 117
Insulin 13, 42, 73
Insulin tolerance test 190-2
Intermediate lobe 5, 12, 136
Internalisation of receptors 65-6
Isotopes 22

Jet-lag 52

Kallman's syndrome 117
Kidney 50, 163
Klinefelter's syndrome 124

Labour 115, 165
Lactation 80-2, 115, 165
Lactotroph 6, 175
Leu-enkephalin 135
Leydig cells 116-17
Limbic system 38
Lipotrophin 29, 135
Luteinising hormone 5, 41, 85
Luteinising hormone releasing hormone (LHRH) 2, 33, 41, 49, 54, 58, 61, 79, 118 *et seq.*
Luteolysis 114
Lysosomes 65
Lysine vasopressin 134, 170

Magnocellular neurones 35, 158
Mamillary bodies 4, 34, 37
Mammary gland 76, 80-1
Mammary strip assay 14, 17-18
Mammotrophs *see* lactotrophs
Mammotropic assay for prolactin 17

Medial forebrain bundle 38
Median eminence 1, 5, 9
Medulla 38
Melanocyte stimulating hormone 29, 135–7
Melatonin 112
Memory 171
Menarche 77, 122
Menopause 115
Menstrual cycle 112–14
Mesencephalon 39
Messenger RNA 53, 64, 72
Met-enkephalin 135
Microadenoma 173
Microfilaments 69
Micropenis 72
Microtubule 69
Milk ejection 3, 164
Mineralocorticoid *see* aldosterone
Monoclonal antibodies 22
Morphine *see* opiates
Multiplication stimulating activity 66, 95
Myxoedema 132, 168

Naloxone 114
Nelson's syndrome 151, 183
Neocortex 38–9
Neural lobe *see* posterior pituitary
Neuroglycopenia 190–1
Neurohypophysis *see* posterior pituitary
Neurointermediate lobe 136
Neuroleptic drugs 81
Neurophysins 155
Neurosarcoidosis 45
Neurosecretion 32, 154
Neurosecretory cells 1, 36, 154
Neurotransmitter 54
Noradrenergic pathway 11, 54, 56, 58, 110, 130
Nuclear receptors 64

Oestradiol 77, 113
Oestrogen 41, 49, 80–1, 83
Oligomenorrhoea 85, 120
Opiates 59
Opioid peptides 60, 80, 141, 156
Optic chiasma 3, 4, 10, 40
Osmolality 158–9
Osmoreceptors 158–9, 169
Ovary 47, 112–14
Ovulation 58, 112–14
Oxytocin 14, 42, 49, 59, 154, 164

Parasympathetic system 32
Parathyroid hormone 18
Pars intermedia *see* intermediate lobe
Pars nervosa *see* posterior pituitary
Pars tuberalis 4, 5

Parturition 115, 165
Paraventricular nucleus 4, 35–7
Pergolide 87–8, 176
Periodic Schiff positive 5
Periventricular nuclei 35
Permeability of the cell 72–3
Permissive action 62
Phosphatidyl inositol 71
Phosphodiesterase 69
Phosphorylase a and b 63, 70
Phosphorylase kinase 63, 69, 72
Pickwickian syndrome 42
Pineal gland 58
Pituicyte 1, 8
    Anatomy 3–5
    Blood supply 9–10
    Embryology 10–12
Polycystic ovary syndrome 85
Polydipsia 32, 34, 168–9
Polyethylene glycol 22
Polysomes 53
Polyuria 42, 168–9
Portal circulation 1, 9–10, 11, 40
Positive feedback 49, 109
Posterior pituitary gland 8–9, 153 *et seq.*
Prader-Willi syndrome 38, 124
Precision 29
Precocious puberty 120, 122
Pregnancy 4, 77, 114–15
Preoptic area 35, 109
Progesterone 80–1, 116
Prohormone 33
Prolactin 7, 12, 23–5, 29, 41, 43, 55, 76–89
Prolactin release inhibiting factor (PIF) 78–80
Prolactinomas 173–82
Pro-opiocortin 5, 53, 136
Protein kinase 63–4, 67
Psychiatric disorder 52, 60
Puberty 43, 62, 111–12
Pulsatile hormone secretion 30, 114, 142

Quality control 24

Radioimmunoassay *see* assay
Rathke's pouch 10, 43
Receptor subunit of protein kinase 67
Receptors membrane 62–8, 71
    sensory 48
Recovery plasma 28
Regulatory protein 67
REM sleep 52
Renal failure 84
Reticular activating system 32
Ribosomes 53

Index

Saturation analysis 19
Schwartz-Barrter syndrome 167
Secretion 13
Second antibody 23-4
Second messenger 53, 62
Secretory granules 53
Sella turcica 3, 11
Seminiferous tubule 116
Separation (bound from free hormone) 22-3
Sep-Paks 26
Septum 38
Septum pellucidum 37
Serotonin *see* 5-hydroxytryptamine
Serotoninergic pathways 54
Sertoli cells 117
Servo mechanisms 48
Sex steroids *see* oestrogen, progesterone, testosterone
Sheehan's syndrome 82
Sleep 77, 92
Somatomedin 65, 94-6
Somatostatin 28, 33, 56, 97-9, 128, 133, 186
Somatotrophs 6
Solid phase system 22
Spermatogenesis 116-17
Sphenoid sinus 4
Spherosil 25
Standard hormone preparations 14
Steroid hormones 64
Stimulus-secretion coupling 158
Stress 30, 82
Stria terminalis 35
Suckling 77, 165
Sulphation factor *see* somatomedin
Suprachiasmatic nucleus 51
Supraoptic nucleus 4, 8, 35, 37
Supraregional Assay Service 30
Surgery 161
Sympathetic nervous system 32

Syndrome of inappropriate vasopressin secretion (SIADH) 60, 167

Tachyphylaxis 66
Tanycytes 39
Temperature regulation 43
Testis 47
Testosterone 86, 115-17
Third ventricle 4, 10, 34
Thirst 169, 199
Thyroid hormones 12, 49, 64
Thyroid stimulating antibodies 74
Thyrotrophin 5, 12, 26, 49, 56, 61, 80, 83
Thyrotrophin releasing hormone 1, 33, 51, 55-6, 61, 79
Thyrotrophs 6
Thyroxine 7, 42, 128, 188
Tibia assay 15
Tracer for assay 20
Tranquillisers 83, 84
Trans-sphenoidal surgery 176-7
Tri-iodothyronine 128
Tuber cinereum 34
Tuberculosis 45, 168
Tuberoinfundibular system 35-7
Tumours 78, 84
 pituitary 3, 7-8, 43, 133
Turner's syndrome 117, 124

Vasoactive intestinal peptide 55
Vasopressin 14, 16, 41, 50, 59, 153 *et seq.*
Visual defect 4, 187
Vitamin D 64
Ventromedial nucleus 91
Volume receptors 162

Weight 124

XO karyotype 117, 124
XXY karyotrope 124